Return to Play Following Musculoskeletal Injury

Editor

BRETT D. OWENS

CLINICS IN SPORTS MEDICINE

www.sportsmed.theclinics.com

Consulting Editor
MARK D. MILLER

October 2016 • Volume 35 • Number 4

ELSEVIER

1600 John F. Kennedy Boulevard • Suite 1800 • Philadelphia, Pennsylvania, 19103-2899

http://www.theclinics.com

CLINICS IN SPORTS MEDICINE Volume 35, Number 4
October 2016 ISSN 0278-5919, ISBN-13: 978-0-323-46335-5

Editor: Jennifer Flynn-Briggs
Developmental Editor: Donald Mumford

Clinics in Sports Medicine (ISSN 0278-5919) is published quarterly by Elsevier Inc., 360 Park Avenue South, New York, NY 10010-1710. Months of issue are January, April, July, and October. Business and Editorial Offices: 1600 John F. Kennedy Blvd., Ste. 1800, Philadelphia, PA 19103-2899. Customer Service Office: 3251 Riverport Lane, Maryland Heights, MO 63043. Periodicals postage paid at New York, NY and additional mailing offices. Subscription prices are $340.00 per year (US individuals), $597.00 per year (US institutions), $100.00 per year (US students), $385.00 per year (Canadian individuals), $737.00 per year (Canadian institutions), $235.00 (Canadian students), $470.00 per year (foreign individuals), $737.00 per year (foreign institutions), and $235.00 per year (foreign students). Foreign air speed delivery is included in all *Clinics* subscription prices. All prices are subject to change without notice. **POSTMASTER:** Send address changes to *Clinics in Sports Medicine*, Elsevier Health Sciences Division, Subscription Customer Service, 3251 Riverport Lane, Maryland Heights, MO 63043. Customer Service (orders, claims, online, change of address): Elsevier Health Sciences Division, Subscription Customer Service, 3251 Riverport Lane, Maryland Heights, MO 63043. **Tel: 1-800-654-2452 (U.S. and Canada); 314-447-8871 (outside U.S. and Canada). Fax: 314-447-8029.** E-mail: **journalscustomerservice-usa@elsevier.com (for print support); journalsonlinesupport-usa@ elsevier.com (for online support).**

Reprints. For copies of 100 or more of articles in this publication, please contact the Commercial Reprints Department, Elsevier Inc., 360 Park Avenue South, New York, NY 10010-1710. Tel.: 212-633-3874; Fax: 212-633-3820; E-mail: reprints@elsevier.com.

Clinics in Sports Medicine is covered in *MEDLINE/PubMed (Index Medicus) Current Contents/Clinical Medicine, Excerpta Medica,* and *ISI/Biomed.*

Contributors

CONSULTING EDITOR

MARK D. MILLER, MD
S. Ward Casscells Professor, Head, Division of Sports Medicine, Department of Orthopaedic Surgery, University of Virginia, Charlottesville, Virginia; Team Physician, James Madison University, Harrisonburg, Virginia

EDITOR

BRETT D. OWENS, MD
Professor of Orthopaedic Surgery, Department of Orthopaedics, Brown Alpert Medical School, Warren Alpert Medical School of Brown University, Providence, Rhode Island

AUTHORS

JEREMY A. ALLAND, MD
Department of Orthopaedic Surgery, Rush University Medical Center, Chicago, Illinois

JUSTIN C. ANDERSON, MD
Orthopedic Surgery Resident, Orthopedic Surgery Service, Department of Surgery, Madigan Army Medical Center, Tacoma, Washington

ROBERT B. ANDERSON, MD
OrthoCarolina Foot and Ankle Institute, Charlotte, North Carolina

ASHEESH BEDI, MD
Harold and Helen W. Gehring Professor of Orthopaedic Surgery, Chief, Sports Medicine and Shoulder Surgery, Domino's Farms – MedSport, University of Michigan Health System, Ann Arbor, Michigan

CPT ALAINA M. BRELIN, MD
Orthopaedic Surgery Department, Walter Reed National Military Medical Center, Bethesda, Maryland

BRIAN BUSCONI, MD
Department of Orthopaedic Surgery, University of Massachusetts, Worcester, Massachusetts

EDWARD LYLE CAIN Jr, MD
Founder and Fellowship Director, Andrews Sports Medicine and Orthopaedic Center, American Sports Medicine Institute, Birmingham, Alabama

PATRICK M. CHASSE, DPT
Department of Physical and Occupational Therapy, Duke Sports Sciences Institute, Duke University, Durham, North Carolina

HO-RIM CHOI, MD
Department of Orthopaedic Surgery, University of Massachusetts, Worcester,
Massachusetts

RALPH W. COOK, BS
Department of Orthopaedic Surgery, Northwestern University Feinberg School of
Medicine, Northwestern University, Chicago, Illinois

MAJ JONATHAN F. DICKENS, MD
Department of Orthopaedic Surgery, Walter Reed National Military Medical Center,
Bethesda, Maryland

VICKIE D. DILLS, PT, DPT
Department of Orthopaedic Surgery, University of Massachusetts, Worcester,
Massachusetts

CPT MICHAEL A. DONOHUE, MD
Department of Orthopaedic Surgery, Walter Reed National Military Medical Center,
Bethesda, Maryland

PETE DRAOVITCH, PT, MS, ATC, CSCS, SCS
Clinical Supervisor, The Hip, James M. Benson Sports Rehabilitation Center, New York,
New York

THEODORA DWORAK, MD
Department of Orthopaedic Surgery, Walter Reed National Military Medical Center,
Bethesda, Maryland

OSAMA ELATTAR, MD
Department of Orthopaedic Surgery, University of Massachusetts, Worcester,
Massachusetts

PAUL D. FADALE, MD
Sports Medicine Fellowship Director; Professor and Chief of Sports Medicine,
Department of Orthopaedics, Warren Alpert Medical School of Brown University,
Providence, Rhode Island

BRADEN C. FLEMING, PhD
Professor, Department of Orthopaedics, Warren Alpert Medical School of Brown
University, Providence, Rhode Island

ANDREA HALIM, MD
Fellow, Division of Hand Surgery, Department of Orthopaedics, Alpert Medical School of
Brown University, Providence, Rhode Island

WELLINGTON K. HSU, MD
Department of Orthopaedic Surgery, Northwestern University Feinberg School of
Medicine, Northwestern University, Chicago, Illinois

MICHAEL J. HULSTYN, MD
Associate Professor, Department of Orthopaedics, Warren Alpert Medical School of
Brown University, Providence, Rhode Island

DANIEL G. KANG, MD
Assistant Professor, Orthopedic Surgery Service, Department of Surgery, Madigan Army
Medical Center, Tacoma, Washington

CHRISTOPHER KIM, MD
Department of Orthopaedic Surgery, Duke Sports Sciences Institute, Duke University, Durham, North Carolina

ANDREW KUHN, BA
Domino's Farms – MedSport, University of Michigan Health System, Ann Arbor, Michigan

SIMON LEE, MD, MPH
Orthopaedic Surgery House Officer, University of Michigan Health System, Ann Arbor, Michigan

RONALD A. LEHMAN Jr, MD
Professor, Department of Orthopedic Surgery, Columbia University Medical Center, The Spine Hospital – New York Presbyterian/The Allen Hospital, New York, New York

COLIN B. McCULLOCH, BA
Department of Orthopaedic Surgery, Rush University Medical Center, Chicago, Illinois

OWEN McGONIGLE, MD
Fellow, Andrews Sports Medicine and Orthopaedic Center, American Sports Medicine Institute, Birmingham, Alabama

RYAN C. MORRIS, DO
Sports Medicine Fellow, Department of Orthopaedics, Warren Alpert Medical School of Brown University, Providence, Rhode Island

BRETT D. OWENS, MD
Professor of Orthopaedic Surgery, Department of Orthopaedics, Brown Alpert Medical School, Warren Alpert Medical School of Brown University, Providence, Rhode Island

ANTHONY ROMEO, MD
Department of Orthopaedic Surgery, Rush University Medical Center, Chicago, Illinois

CDR JOHN-PAUL H. RUE, MD
Orthopaedic Surgery Department, Walter Reed National Military Medical Center, Bethesda, Maryland

SCOTT B. SHAWEN, MD
Associate Professor, Uniformed Services University of the Health Sciences, Bethesda, Maryland; OrthoCarolina Foot and Ankle Institute, Charlotte, North Carolina

DEAN C. TAYLOR, MD
Department of Orthopaedic Surgery, Duke Sports Sciences Institute, Duke University, Durham, North Carolina

ROBERT THORSNESS, MD
Department of Orthopaedic Surgery, Rush University Medical Center, Chicago, Illinois

ARNOLD-PETER C. WEISS, MD
R. Scot Sellers Scholar of Hand Surgery, Vice Chairman and Professor of Orthopaedics, Division of Hand Surgery, Department of Orthopaedics, Alpert Medical School of Brown University, Providence, Rhode Island

Contents

Criteria for return to sports and athletic activities after cervical spine surgery are unclear. There is limited literature regarding the outcomes and
optimal criteria. Determining return to play criteria remains a challenge
and continues to depend on the experience and good judgment of the
treating surgeon. There is strong consensus in the literature, despite lack
of evidence-based data, that athletes after single-level anterior cervical
discectomy and fusion (ACDF) may safely return to collision and high-
velocity sports. The athlete should be counseled and managed on a
case-by-case basis, taking into consideration the type of sport, player-
specific variables, and type of surgery performed.

Anterior shoulder instability in athletes may lead to time lost from participation and decreases in level of play. Contact, collision, and overhead athletes are at a higher risk than others. Athletes may successfully be
returned to play but operative stabilization should be considered for
long-term treatment of recurrent instability. Open and arthroscopic stabilization procedures for athletes with less than 20% to 25% bone loss
improve return to play rates and decrease recurrent instability, with a
slightly lower recurrence with open stabilization. For athletes with greater
than 20% to 25% bone loss, an open osseous augmentation procedure
should be considered.

The throwing athlete's shoulder is a unique, complex entity with challenges
in diagnosis and management. The shoulders in these athletes possess
unique biomechanics and pathologic conditions. Unfortunately, return to
play outcomes are often poor when specifically evaluating overhead athletes, especially with regard to SLAP repair. It is imperative for the surgeon
to be cautious when indicating these athletes for surgery, because
although they may demonstrate improvements in pain and general function, subtle changes in accuracy or velocity as a result of surgery can

significantly affect the success of an overhead throwing athlete at the competitive level.

Ulnar collateral ligament injury in the overhead athlete typically presents as activity-related pain with loss of velocity and control. Treatment options range from nonoperative rehabilitation to ligament reconstruction. Surgical reconstruction is frequently required to allow the athlete to return to competition and many surgical techniques have been described. The rehabilitation process to return back to overhead athletics, in particular pitching, is prolonged and requires progression through multiple phases. Despite this, surgical treatment has been shown by multiple investigators to be successful at returning athletes to their previous level of competition.

Wrist and hand injuries are common among athletes, and can lead to considerable disability. Dislocations and soft tissue injuries are common and require prompt recognition and treatment. Accurate diagnosis and early immobilization are often key to getting players back to their sport early. Some injuries require surgery; operative intervention allows the player to return to their sport more quickly or with less long-term disability. This article discusses the spectrum of injury from distal radius fractures to mallet fingers, and offers some general guidelines for the surgeon in how to counsel and treat athletes with these problems.

Surgical management of lumbar spine conditions can produce excellent outcomes in athletes. Microdiscectomy for lumbar disc herniation has favorable outcomes; most athletes return to play at preoperative performance levels. Direct pars repair is successful in younger athletes, with high rates of return to play for a variety of fixation techniques. Fusion in athletes with scoliosis is a negative predictor. There are few evidence-based return to play criteria. Athletes should demonstrate full resolution of symptoms and flexibility, endurance, and strength before returning to play. Deciding when to return an athlete to sport depends on particular injury sustained, sport, and individual factors.

Sports hernia is a condition that causes acute/chronic pain of low abdominal, groin, or adductor area in athletes. It is considered a weakness in the rectus abdominis insertion or posterior inguinal wall of lower abdomen caused by acute or repetitive injury of the structure. It is most commonly seen in soccer, ice hockey, and martial arts players who require acute cutting, pivoting, or kicking. A variety of surgical options have been reported with successful outcome and with high rates of return to the sports in a majority of cases.

Femoroacetabular impingement may be particularly disabling to the high-demand athlete, especially those with significant cutting and pivoting requirements. If nonoperative treatment fails to adequately alleviate symptoms or sufficiently restore function in the athlete, hip arthroscopy can lead to improved pain, improved range of motion, and high rates of return to play with proper postoperative rehabilitation. The rate of return to previous level of competition is also high with accurate diagnosis and well-executed correction of deformity. A clear understanding of the etiology, diagnosis, management, and outcomes is essential for clinicians to optimally help patients to return to play.

Anterior cruciate ligament reconstructions are commonly performed in an attempt to return an athlete to sports activities. Accelerated rehabilitation has made recovery for surgery more predictable and shortened the timeline for return to play. Despite success with and advancements in anterior cruciate ligament reconstructions, some athletes still fail to return to play.

Meniscus tears are commonly encountered in the athletic population and can result in significant loss of playing time. Current treatment methods for acute tears consist of meniscectomy and meniscal repair, whereas meniscal allograft transplant is reserved as a salvage procedure for symptomatic meniscectomized patients who desire a more functional knee. This review describes the postoperative rehabilitation protocol for each procedure and evaluates the outcomes in existing literature as it pertains to the athlete.

Medial collateral ligament injuries are common in the athletic population. Partial injuries are treated nonoperatively with excellent outcomes. Complete ruptures may be treated nonoperatively, although some will require surgery. A comprehensive rehabilitation program is critical to outcome, but a standardized program for all injuries does not exist. Most of the literature regarding nonoperative and postoperative rehabilitation include observational reports and case studies. Level I studies comparing rehabilitation protocols have not been published. The goal of the injured athlete is to not only return to play with no functional limitations, but to also address risk factors and prevent future injuries.

Scott B. Shawen, Theodora Dworak, and Robert B. Anderson

Ankle sprains are the most common musculoskeletal injury occurring during athletics. Proper initial treatment with supportive pain control, limited immobilization, early return to weight bearing and range of motion, and directed physical therapy are essential for preventing recurrent injury. Reconstruction of the lateral ligaments is indicated for patients with continued instability and dysfunction despite physical therapy. Return to athletic activity should be reserved for athletes who have regained strength, proprioception, and range of motion of the injured ankle. Athletes with a history of an ankle sprain should be prophylactically braced or tapped to reduce risk of recurrent injury.

CLINICS IN SPORTS MEDICINE

RELATED INTEREST

Orthopedic Clinics, July 2016 (Vol. 47, Issue 3)
Orthopedic Urgencies and Emergencies
James H. Calandruccio, Benjamin J. Grear, Benjamin M. Mauck, Jeffrey R. Sawyer,
Patrick C. Toy, and John C. Weinlein, *Editors*
Available at: http://www.orthopedic.theclinics.com/

THE CLINICS ARE AVAILABLE ONLINE!
Access your subscription at:
www.theclinics.com

RELATED INTEREST

Foreword

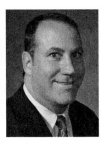

Mark D. Miller, MD
Consulting Editor

This issue addresses a question that resonates in locker rooms, training rooms, clinics, and coaches' offices. As physicians, we should add another word to this age-old question: When can the athlete *safely* return to play? Dr Brett Owens, who has plenty of experience in this area, first at West Point and now in the Ivy League, has taken on this challenge and presents it here, in a literally head-to-toe approach. He has assembled an impressive group of team physicians and surgeons to provide recommendations for a variety of injuries and surgeries. Because there is often little guidance in the literature on this important question, they have often "gone out on a limb" to provide these recommendations. Although the focus of this issue is on musculoskeletal injuries, we need to be mindful of return-to-play guidelines for a variety of medical conditions as well. In light of recent research and media attention, I would like to remind the readers that return to play after concussion includes the principle that the athlete should NEVER return to play the same day following a concussion.

I hope that this issue will be of use to team physicians at all levels and for all sports. I congratulate and sincerely thank Dr Brett Owens and all of the authors that participated in this issue on "Return to Play."

Mark D. Miller, MD
Division of Sports Medicine
Department of Orthopaedic Surgery
University of Virginia
Miller Review Course
400 Ray C. Hunt Drive, Suite 330
Charlottesville, VA 22908-0159, USA

E-mail address:
mdm3p@virginia.edu

Clin Sports Med 35 (2016) xiii
http://dx.doi.org/10.1016/j.csm.2016.06.002
0278-5919/16/$ – see front matter © 2016 Published by Elsevier Inc.

sportsmed.theclinics.com

Preface

Return to Play Following Musculoskeletal Injury

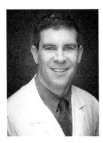

Brett D. Owens, MD
Editor

It's not whether you get knocked down, it's whether you get up.
—*Vince Lombardi*

In my professional life, I have experienced few things as challenging or rewarding as taking care of athletes. From youth and recreational participants to professional and Olympic athletes, those competing at all levels of sport expect the highest levels of performance and continually push the envelope of care. They force those who care for them to continually challenge the conventional wisdom and advance diagnostic and treatment timelines and protocols. The advances seen with the treatment of high-level athletes has a "trickle-down" effect on the care of weekend warriors. And while the management of these populations is different, the entire field is propelled by these advances, all born out of the drive to return to play. I have learned so much from my patients and continue to do so.

Central to caring for athletes is the concept of "return to play." Athletes need and want to know about the long-term ramifications of their injury and treatment decisions. However, the first question is ALWAYS, "Doc, when can I play again?" With some injuries, there is substantial literature to help guide clinicians in making this prognosis; however, some injuries and conditions present challenges due to sparse published reports. Many surgical outcomes studies comprise combined athlete and nonathlete populations and focus on patient-reported outcomes or clinician evaluation, but make little mention of the critical first question of the athlete. This special issue has been developed with this central question in mind. We have assembled an impressive group of experts in their respective fields and asked them to present a concise review of the literature and their approach to surgical and rehabilitation treatment of specific injuries in athletes and return to play considerations. We hope this information will help

Clin Sports Med 35 (2016) xv–xvi
http://dx.doi.org/10.1016/j.csm.2016.06.001
0278-5919/16/$ – see front matter © 2016 Published by Elsevier Inc.

sportsmed.theclinics.com

clinicians who care for athletes prepare to answer that critical first question: "Doc, when can I play again?"

Brett D. Owens, MD
Professor of Orthopaedic Surgery
Department of Orthopaedics
Brown Alpert Medical School
100 Butler Drive
Providence, RI 02906, USA

E-mail address:
owensbrett@gmail.com

Return to Play After Cervical Disc Surgery

Daniel G. Kang, MD[a], Justin C. Anderson, MD[a], Ronald A. Lehman Jr, MD[b],*

KEYWORDS

- Cervical disc surgery • Anterior cervical discectomy and fusion • Return to play
- Spinal cord injury • Spinal cord contusion • Spinal stenosis • Cervical disc herniation
- Cervical spondylosis

KEY POINTS

- Criteria for return to play after cervical disc surgery are unclear, with limited literature consisting mostly of case reports and small retrospective series.
- There is strong consensus in the literature, despite a lack of evidence-based data, that athletes after single-level anterior cervical discectomy and fusion (ACDF) may safely return to collision and high-velocity sports.
- Controversy remains regarding return to play after 2- and 3-level ACDF constructs, with most studies recommending relative contraindication for return to collision and high-velocity sports.
- Return to play after other surgical treatment options, such as cervical disc arthroplasty, posterior cervical laminoforaminotomy, and posterior cervical laminaplasty, remains unclear.
- Decision making for return to play remains a challenge and continues to depend on the experience and good judgment of the treating surgeon.

INTRODUCTION

Criteria for return to sports and athletic activities after cervical spine surgery are unclear, and remain a challenging topic given the potential catastrophic consequences. Cervical disc disease can impact significantly the careers of professional or elite

No outside funding sources were used for this study. The authors have no conflicts of interest related to this work. No reproduced copyrighted materials.

The opinions or assertions contained herein are the private views of the authors and are not to be construed as official or as reflecting the views of the United States Army or the Department of Defense. One or more authors are employees of the United States government. This work was prepared as part of their official duties and as such, there is no copyright to be transferred.

[a] Orthopedic Surgery Service, Department of Surgery, Madigan Army Medical Center, 9040 Jackson Avenue, Tacoma, WA 98431, USA; [b] Department of Orthopedic Surgery, Columbia University Medical Center, The Spine Hospital – New York Presbyterian/The Allen Hospital, 5141 Broadway, 3 Field West, New York, NY 10034, USA
* Corresponding author.
E-mail address: ronaldalehman@yahoo.com

Clin Sports Med 35 (2016) 529–543
http://dx.doi.org/10.1016/j.csm.2016.05.001   **sportsmed.theclinics.com**
0278-5919/16/$ – see front matter Published by Elsevier Inc.

athletes, particularly those involved in collision or high-velocity sports.[1,2] Although most athletes with acute cervical disc herniation or degenerative disc disease can be treated nonoperatively,[3] those with persistent or progressive symptoms may require operative intervention. The spine surgeon may experience substantial pressure from the patient, family members, and coaching and athletic staff to provide recommendations on the timing, prognosis, and potential recovery after cervical disc surgery.[4] Unfortunately, there is limited literature, consisting mostly of case reports and small retrospective series, regarding the outcomes and optimal return to play criteria after cervical disc surgery. Therefore, recommendations are often arbitrary, based on the good judgment and the experience of the treating surgeon.[4] Although inadequate rehabilitation or imprudent return to play may cause suboptimal outcomes after some orthopedic procedures, the most feared and serious complication after cervical spine surgery is paralysis. Even in athletes without previous surgery, catastrophic spinal cord injury (SCI) from cervical spine fracture or injury remains an inherent risk during collision and high-velocity sports,[4,5] and whether this risk is increased after cervical disc surgery is unknown. Given the lack of evidence-based recommendations for return to play in athletes after cervical disc surgery, this review provides a summary of the reported outcomes and available recommendations. We set out to review the available return to play criteria and guidelines comprehensively, to allow the spine surgeon and athlete to assess the potential risks and make the most informed decision in this unique patient population.

EPIDEMIOLOGY OF CERVICAL SPONDYLOSIS IN THE GENERAL POPULATION

Cervical spondylosis is a common entity that increases with age, and is a common cause of clinic visits, health care resource use, and reduction in quality of life.[6] Up to 10% of the general population will experience neck pain at any given time,[7] and a retrospective population-based review found the average annual incidence of cervical radiculopathy per 100,000 people to be 107.3 for men and 63.5 for women.[3] Cervical disc protrusion was responsible for radiculopathy in 21.9% of these patients, whereas 68.4% was attributed to spondylosis, disc protrusion, or both.[3]

Autopsy studies have shown that cervical disc degeneration has a prevalence of 10% in the third decade of life and approaches 96% by the eighth decade.[8] Similarly, a landmark study by Boden and colleagues[9] found that MRI of asymptomatic individuals demonstrated degenerative changes in 25% of patients younger than 40 years of age and 60% of patients older than 40 years. Other studies have demonstrated that persons older than age 60 have degenerative changes on lateral cervical radiographs in more than 60% to 75% of persons and MRI changes in more than 85% of asymptomatic individuals.[6,10,11] These studies of asymptomatic patients with radiographic or MRI findings of cervical spondylosis demonstrate the relatively poor correlation between the presence of imaging findings and clinical manifestations of foraminal or central stenosis.

EPIDEMIOLOGY OF CERVICAL SPONDYLOSIS IN ATHLETES

Although cervical spondylosis is common in the general population, it follows an age-related curve and is thus a less frequent problem in the younger athletic population.[12] However, sports participation exposes the cervical spine in young athletes to theoretic risk factors not seen in the general population, and specifically long-term participation in collision sports seems to increase the risk of radiographic cervical spondylosis.[1,6,13–16] Cumulative effects of repetitive, high-intensity loading on the spinal column, as occurs during some collision sports, may result in the propagation and development of disc bulges, disc degeneration, spinal osteophytes, and ligamentum flavum hypertrophy, causing symptoms such as foraminal and central stenosis.[6,13,17–22] In contrast, high-performance athletes participating in noncontact sports may actually be protected against the development of such disease.[15] Some postulate that increased support from the surrounding musculature in the noncontact athlete off-loads the cervical spine and reduces progression of disc disease.[6,15]

In the United States, National Football League (NFL) players are a group of elite athletes who have generated interest on the long-term musculoskeletal impact of high-energy collision sports. In a study of retired NFL players aged 30 to 49 years, 36.6% reported that they had been diagnosed with arthritis of the neck, compared with only 16.9% of age-matched controls.[23] In addition, cervical canal stenosis from spondylosis with osteophyte formation, herniated disc, congenital narrowing of the canal, or any combination of these elements is estimated to be 7 per 10,000 football participants.[24]

Gray and colleagues[25] found from 2000 to 2012 that there were a total of 275 disc herniations in the NFL, which accounted for 13% of all spine injuries and 6% of all cervical spine injuries. The majority of disc herniations occurred in the lumbar region (74%), followed next by the cervical region (23%). Cervical herniations resulted in the most lost practice time by region (cervical, thoracic, lumbar) at a mean of 113 practices and a median of 24 practices missed per cervical disc herniation. The most common mechanisms leading to cervical disc herniation were tackling (31%) and blocking (25%), and subsequently linebackers (18%) and defensive backs (16%) had the highest number of cervical herniations.

In another study of NFL players, Mall and colleagues[5] found over an 11-season time period that 7% of total injuries had occurred in the axial skeleton. Nearly one-half (44.7%) of these injuries occurred in the cervical spine, and cervical injuries lead to an average of 23.4 days missed per injury. Of the 987 documented injuries to the cervical spine, there were 453 nerve injuries (45.9%), 214 muscular injuries (21.7%), 153 sprains (5.5%), 57 injuries to the disc (5.8%), and 46 impingement syndromes (4.7%).[5] The authors also found tackling and, to a lesser extent blocking, were the actions most strongly associated with injury to the cervical spine.[5,26]

Although American football and high school wrestling athletes sustain the highest rates of cervical spine injuries in the United States,[27] rugby is a collision sport more popular outside the United States and front-row rugby players have been found to experience high rates of cervical degeneration.[28–30] In 1 study, among a group of 101 former rugby players and 85 matched controls, there were significantly more rugby players who complained of chronic neck pain (50.50% vs 31.76%, respectively).[29]

RISK OF SPINAL CORD INJURY DURING SPORTS

The most devastating and feared cervical spine injury in collision sports is catastrophic SCI, and typically results from cervical spine fractures, fracture dislocations, and traumatic disc herniations.[6] The most frequent injuries, however, are cervical cord neuropraxia and unilateral brachial plexus or cervical root neuropraxias, termed "stingers" and "burners,"[31] which are generally self-limiting and do not require intervention. Despite the high-profile media attention, SCI resulting in quadriplegia is extremely rare during most popular sports. There were a total of 10,047 reported SCIs in the United States in 2014.[32] Sports injuries were the fourth most common cause of SCI between 2010 and 2014 (9.0%), after vehicular accidents (37.7%), falls (30.6%), and violence (13.8%). The most frequently reported sports-related SCI in 2014 was diving accidents (6.0%)[33]; however, these typically occur among recreational, inexperienced divers.[34] Other commonly reported sports-related SCIs include football, rugby, skiing, winter sports, horseback riding, surfing, wrestling, gymnastics, field sports, and water skiing.[32]

Because of the popularity of American football in the United States, cervical spine injuries have been characterized most frequently in this athlete population and have become the topic of much concern.[19] In a study of high school and college football players over a 13-year period, Boden and colleagues[35] identified 76 injuries resulting in quadriplegia for a mean annual incidence of 0.52 per 100,000 participants. The incidence at the college level was 1.65 times higher than the high school incidence.[35] Most of the injuries were suffered by players on defense (63.4%), with the greatest percentage of injuries occurring to defensive backs (44.3%). The activity at the time of injury was determined to be making a tackle in 79.7% of injuries.[35] It has been suggested that defensive backs are most susceptible to SCI because of the frequency at which they must make tackles and the split-second decisions they must make to be effective in making tackles of the opposing receivers.[1]

Similar studies have been conducted in Canadian hockey players.[36] From 1943 to 2011, 355 spinal injuries in hockey players have been documented. Of the cases with sufficient documentation, it was determined that the majority of cases (61.2%) were SCI with permanent deficits.[36] However, when the data from 2006 to 2011 were analyzed, it was determined that only 9.1% were considered to fall into this severe category. The most common mode of injury was being pushed or checked from behind causing neck hyperextension (35.5%).[36] Hockey organizations have implemented rules against checking from behind to help reduce the frequency of such injuries, although the impact of these new rules is yet to be determined.

LITERATURE REVIEW OF OUTCOMES AND RETURN TO PLAY AFTER CERVICAL DISC SURGERY

As noted, there is limited literature with no randomized studies or large multicenter studies comparing treatment methods, outcomes, or return to play criteria in athletes after cervical disc surgery. Relatively few professional athletes require cervical spine surgery during their active career; therefore, the strongest available literature is likely to remain small, retrospective series with limited outcomes data.[19,37] We provide a review of available studies evaluating the outcomes and return to play after cervical disc surgery in athlete, summarized in **Table 1**.

Hsu[1] in 2011 used team injury reports and newspaper archives, and identified 99 NFL players with a diagnosis of cervical disc herniation (53 operative, and 46 nonoperative). Players who were treated operatively successfully returned to play at a higher rate than those treated nonoperatively. None of the players who returned to play suffered further SCI. Players treated operatively demonstrated a statistically significant greater number of games and years played compared with those treated nonoperatively. Defensive backs, in particular, had significantly poorer outcomes.

In another study, Schroeder and colleagues[2] identified 143 athletes at the NFL level from 2003 to 2011 with a preexisting cervical spine diagnosis. Athletes with a cervical spine diagnosis were less likely to be drafted, had a decreased total number of games played, and decreased career length when compared with those without a cervical spine diagnosis. However, there were no differences in the number of games started and performance score. Seven of the 9 players with a history of cervical spine surgery (4 anterior cervical discectomy and fusion [ACDF], 2 foraminotomies, and 1 suboccipital craniectomy with C1 laminectomy) were drafted and had no differences in career length or performance score when compared with matched controls. No athlete with stenosis or a history of surgery suffered permanent neurologic injury.

Meredith and colleagues[26] studied a total of 16 NFL players with MRI-proven cervical disc herniation with concordant symptoms. Three players underwent 1-level ACDF after failed nonoperative therapy, but only one of these players returned to play. Thirteen players were treated nonoperatively and 8 returned to sport. Of the 5 patients who did not return to sports after nonoperative treatment, 2 patients had evidence of cord compression with cord signal change on MRI and retired rather than undergo surgery, and 3 were released by the teams despite being medically cleared. There were no subsequent SCI in any of the players. The authors concluded that NFL players can safely return to play after the treatment of cervical disc herniation.

Maroon and colleagues[38] reached a similar conclusion, namely, that return to play is safe after cervical disc surgery in elite football players, but postulated that there may be an increased risk for adjacent level disease. The authors reviewed 5 elite football players (4 professional, 1 collegiate) requiring surgery after experiencing episodes of cervical cord neuropraxia. All players underwent single level ACDF with plating, except in 1 case without plating. All 5 athletes returned to play after symptomatic resolution and evidence of solid interbody fusion, ranging from 9 weeks to 8 months postoperatively. Two of the players developed recurrent career-ending disc herniations at adjacent levels: one after 27 games who subsequently underwent adjacent level ACDF, and the other after 7 games who did not undergo surgery. The other 3 players remained asymptomatic throughout the follow-up period, and no athlete suffered permanent neurologic injury.

Another study by Maroon and colleagues[37] reported on 15 professional athletes after a 1-level ACDF by a single neurosurgeon. Thirteen of the 15 athletes returned to their sport at mean of 6 months postoperatively (range, 2–12 months). The 2 players who never returned to play were cleared from a neurologic standpoint, but chose to retire because of an accumulation of multiple orthopedic injuries throughout their careers. During the follow-up period, 5 athletes retired for return to play duration ranging between 1 and 3 years of full participation. Two football players retired after sustaining disc herniations adjacent to their original fusion levels, and 1 wrestler chose to retire secondary to persistent, chronic neck pain without findings of radiculopathy on examination. The authors concluded that athletes may return to play in contact sports after 1-level ACDF, but were concerned there may be an increased risk of adjacent segment disease above or below the level of the fusion.

Andrews and colleagues[28] studied 19 professional rugby union players who underwent ACDF between 1998 and 2003. The most common position was front row forward (n = 13). Thirteen players returned to their previous level of play, 1 returned at a lower level of play, and 5 did not return to play. Nine of the 13 returned to rugby 6 months after the operation, and only 1 player took longer than 12 months to return. Of the players who returned to play, 2 had a recurrence of symptoms, but neither suffered permanent neurologic injury. Patients unable to return to play were limited by persistent pain and/or development of adjacent segment disease. The authors concluded that return to contact sports for their rugby players seemed safe and reasonable.

In contrast with NFL and rugby players, Roberts and colleagues[14] studied 11 Major League Baseball pitchers with cervical disc herniation from 1984 to 2009. Eight pitchers were treated operatively, 7 underwent ACDF, and 1 underwent cervical disk replacement. Eight of the 11 pitchers (73%) returned to play at an average time of 11.6 months after last game played, but those treated with surgery returned to play at a higher rate than those treated nonoperatively (88% vs 33%, respectively). After treatment, average career length was 63 games over 3.7 years, and pitchers had

Table 1
Summary of literature review on return to play after cervical disc surgery

Study	Patients by Sport	Outcome Measures	Cohorts	Results
Schroeder et al,[2] 2014	Football (n = 143)	Successful draft, games played, games started, career length, performance score	Preexisting cervical spine pathology vs no diagnosis	Patients with pathology were less likely to be drafted (65.5% vs 78.1%), had a decreased number of games (42.1 vs 55.6), and had a decreased career length (3.7 vs 4.6 y). In subgroup analysis of the most common diagnoses, only athletes with spondylosis had a decrease in career length, games played, and performance score compared with matched controls. Stenosis and CDH demonstrated no differences. Operative patients drafted had no difference in career length or performance score.
Meredith et al,[26] 2013	Football (n = 16)	Successful return to play	Operative (ACDF) vs nonoperative treatment	Two-thirds of operative patients return to play. Two-thirds of ESI patients return to play. Eight of 13 nonoperative patients return to play.
Maroon et al,[37] 2013	Football (n = 7), wrestling (n = 8)	Successful return to play, time to return to play, recurrence	Operative (ACDF)	Thirteen of 15 athletes return to play between 2 and 12 mo (mean, 6 mo). Two retired because of multiple orthopedic injuries. Five athletes retired for a mean return to play of 1–3 y. Two retired for CDH adjacent to fusion, 1 for chronic neck pain.
Roberts et al,[14] 2011	Baseball (n = 11)	Successful return to play, time to return to play, career length, performance-based (innings, ERA, WHIP)	Operative (ACDF, CDR) vs nonoperative treatment	Seventy-three percent of pitchers return to play at mean 11.6 mo after diagnosis. Operative patients return to play at higher rate (88% vs 33%). Average career postoperatively: 63 games over 3.7 y. Significantly fewer innings pitched per season postoperatively (41.7) compared with preoperatively (68.5).

Study	Sport	Outcome Measures	Comparison	Results
Hsu,[1] 2011	Football (n = 99)	Successful return to play, games played, career length	Operative (ACDF, foraminotomy, indeterminate) vs nonoperative	Seventy-two percent of operative patients vs 46% nonoperative patients successfully return to play. Operative patients played in more games (29.3 vs 14.7) and for more years (2.8 vs 1.5) after treatment vs nonoperative patients.
Andrews et al,[28] 2008	Rugby (n = 19)	Successful return to play, time to return to play, recurrence	Operative (ACDF)	Thirteen of 19 players successfully return to play; 9 of the 13 returned <6 mo postoperatively. Two of 13 who returned had recurrence of symptoms.
Brigham & Capo,[39] 2013	Football (n = 3), basketball (n = 1)	Successful return to play, time to return to play, recurrence	Operative (ACDF)	All athletes successfully return to play: 1 at 5 mo, 1 at 6 mo, 2 the following season. Two of 4 developed new spinal contusions (1/2 adjacent to fusion).
Maroon et al,[38] 2007	Football (n = 5)	Successful return to play, time to return to play, recurrence	Operative (ACDF ± plating)	All athletes successfully return to play from 9 wk to 8 mo postoperatively. Two of 5 developed recurrent career-ending CDH at levels adjacent to fusion.
Saigal et al,[40] 2014	Football (n = 32), soccer (n = 14), baseball/softball (n = 11), basketball (n = 12), martial arts (n = 5), tennis (n = 5), track and field (n = 5), hockey (n = 5), volleyball (n = 3), wrestling (n = 4), other (n = 15)	Successful return to play, time to return to play	Operative spine; instrumented vs noninstrumented spine	Eighty-nine percent of patients with operative spine lesions successfully return to play. Thirty-seven percent of operative spine patients return to play at 1–3 mo; 35% at 3–6 mo. Noninstrumented spine patients return to play significantly more often (97%) than instrumented spine patients (72%).
Gray et al,[25] 2013	Football (n = 275 disc herniations)	Time lost from play	Cervical vs thoracic vs lumbar disc herniations	Twenty-three percent of disc herniations occurred in the cervical spine. CDH resulted in the most lost practice time by region: mean of 113 practices, median of 24 practices.

Abbreviations: ACDF, anterior cervical discectomy and fusion; CDH, cervical disc herniation; CDR, cervical disc replacement; ERA, earned run average; ESI, epidural steroid injection; WHIP, walks and hits per inning pitched.
Data from Refs.[1,2,14,25,26,28,37–40]

significantly fewer average innings pitched per season (41.7 ± 43.1) compared with before treatment (68.5 ± 44.7). For those pitchers treated operatively, there was no difference in performance-based outcomes from before injury to after the operation.

Brigham and Capo[39] reviewed 4 professional athletes (3 NFL players, 1 National Basketball Association player) with documented cervical cord contusions treated with 1- and 2-level ACDF. All 4 athletes had cervical canal stenosis, defined as a lack of functional reserve of CSF surrounding the cord on MRI. One football player returned to play 5 months later, another 6 months later, and the remaining 2 athletes returned to play the season after their surgery. Two athletes developed new contusions: one occurred more than 5 years after surgery and adjacent to his prior fusion, and the other 2 years after surgery. No athlete suffered permanent neurologic injury.

In one of the largest reviews to date, Saigal and colleagues[40] evaluated 189 athletes with structural neurosurgical lesions (118 operative and 71 nonoperative/incidental) reported to the American Academy of Neurologic Surgeons. In the operative treatment group, 89% of athletes returned to play. Of those who returned, 6% returned at 0 to 1 month postoperatively, 37% at 1 to 3 months, 35% at 3 to 6 months, and 22% at 6 months to 1 year. Patients who were instrumented were significantly less likely to successfully return to play than those not instrumented. Of those that successfully return to play, noninstrumented patients returned faster than those instrumented. There was 1 reported patient with cervical disc herniation who underwent ACDF and returned to play between 6 months to 1 year after surgery, but developed a second cervical disc herniation that did not require further surgery.

RETURN TO PLAY CRITERIA AFTER CERVICAL DISC SURGERY

Most patients undergoing cervical disc surgery are not professional athletes, and the decision for return to play in recreational, high school, or nonelite college athletes is typically to retire from collision or high-velocity sports.[19] In the elite high school or college athlete, counseling about the potential risks with return to play should also include a realistic assessment of the athlete's potential to obtain a collegiate scholarship or become professional.[39] There are significantly greater pressures and complex factors for elite and professional athletes when considering surgical treatment of the cervical spine.[37] Elite and professional athletes train for many years for the opportunity to earn a livelihood with their athletic abilities, and most have a relatively brief window of time for their careers.[39] Therefore, other factors that may come into play include nonmedical issues, such as loss of significant pay or contracts, medical liability and workers' compensation issues, and outside influences from the media, coaches, team management, and player representatives.[26,37] The elite or professional athlete, therefore, may be more willing to accept some degree of risk when there is potential for substantial financial gain by returning to play, even at a reduced level.[19] Additionally, high-profile professional athletes often receive consultation from multiple surgeons when considering surgical treatment of a symptomatic cervical disc herniation or cervical spondylosis.[1] Consequently, professional athletes may receive conflicting opinions concerning surgical approach and postoperative return to play clearance criteria from different expert surgeons, which is driven by the limited longitudinal outcomes data and large differences in repetitive stresses and loads during training/competition between different sports.[1,6,37,41] The following discussion focuses on return to play criteria after cervical disc surgery for elite and professional athletes participating in collision and high-velocity sports, because these sports are perceived to hold the greatest risk for further injury. Although guidelines have been recommended previously by some studies on return to play after cervical disc surgery, there remains limited consensus on the optimal implementation. Despite these challenges, surgeons caring for professional and elite athletes are expected to address questions in this unique patient population, and should have an understanding of the current controversies and factors affecting return to play criteria.[6] Decision making for return to play for professional athletes after cervical spine surgery is complex and should be based on the type of sport, patient's underlying diagnosis, objective anatomic considerations from clinical examination and imaging studies, type of surgical procedure, individual response to surgery, and postoperative recovery.[4,37]

Risk Stratification: Type of Sport

Potential risk factors for return to play are not well-defined because, as mentioned, each sport has unique loads and mechanisms related to cervical injury making comparison difficult. Therefore, some studies have recommended categorization of sports based on a perceived gradation of risk. Although specific sports are mentioned, the treating surgeon may increase or decrease the risk category based on their personal experience and good clinical judgment[6,42–44] **(Table 2)**.

The hierarchy of risk as described by Morganti and colleagues[42] is arbitrary, and should be used to help interpret results from the limited available literature based on various types of sports and to provide a framework for counseling athletes on a case-by-case basis.[6] Collision sports are perceived to have the highest risk for injury owing to the frequency of repetitive loading, as well as the large potential loads and energy transfer to the cervical spine.[6] Most contact and high-velocity sports may be considered medium risk; however, these groups of athletes have not been studied as widely as collision athletes and may be at similar risk for cervical injury.[42,44,45] For noncontact sports, the risk for catastrophic injury is very low, and return to play can typically be recommended with appropriate counseling and rehabilitation after cervical disc surgery.[6]

Risk Stratification: Type of Surgery

In addition to the type of sport, an important factor for return to play is the type of surgery performed. Cervical surgery, by itself, is not considered an absolute contraindication to return to play for collision or high-velocity sports.[6,37] ACDF is a well-established surgical option for treatment of symptomatic acute cervical disc herniation and/or cervical spondylosis, but athletes should be followed by a surgeon with expertise in the evaluation of subtle neurologic deficiencies, and who understands the radiographic criteria and postoperative management of cervical spine fusion.[6,37,39] Also, the

---

Table 2
Classification of type of sport with hierarchy of risk

Risk Category	Sport Type	Sports
High risk	Collision	Football, ice hockey, rugby, martial arts, wrestling
Medium risk	Contact	Lacrosse, soccer, basketball, volleyball, baseball, water polo
	Noncontact, high velocity	Skiing, gymnastics, cheerleading
Low risk	Noncontact, repetitive load	Running, tennis, Olympic lifting, functional fitness
	Noncontact, low impact	Swimming, cycling, golf, bowling, rowing

Adapted from Morganti C, Sweeney CA, Albanese SA, et al. Return to play after cervical spine injury. Spine 2001;26:1131–6.

presence of long tract signs are known to be normal findings in asymptomatic individuals, such as positive Hoffman sign (10%) or inverted radial reflex (25%), and should not be taken out of context with the clinical examination and imaging findings.[39,46]

Overall, there is reasonable consensus in the literature that elite and professional athletes may safely return to collision and high-velocity sports after single-level subaxial ACDF using modern anterior plating techniques[1,4,19,28,37,39,42,47–51] (Box 1). The first guidelines for return to play of athletes with fused cervical segments was by Torg and Ramsey-Emrhein[51] in 1997. The authors discuss management of patients with Klippel–Feil syndrome with 1- or 2-level subaxial cervical segments congenitally fused, and recommended no contraindications for return to play in the presence of full cervical range of motion and no occipital–cervical anomalies or instability.[19,47]

However, controversy remains surrounding athletes who have undergone multilevel ACDF, with most studies recommending relative contraindication for return to collision and high-velocity sports after both 2- and 3-level constructs.[34,38,52] Torg and colleagues[53] recommended 2- or 3-level fusion constructs present a relative contraindication for return to play, whereas a 4-level or more anterior or posterior fusion presents an absolute contraindication for return to play. In contrast, Burnett and colleagues recommended that constructs with 3 or more levels be excluded permanently from collision and contact sports. The main concern of these authors was increased junctional stresses with longer fusion constructs and the increased risk of adjacent segment degeneration and disease.[37] Regardless of fusion length, all athletes after ACDF should be counseled on the inherent risk of adjacent segment degeneration and disease above or below the fused levels,[37–39] with the C3-C4 level being identified in some studies as having a propensity to develop problems.[22,39]

The criteria for return to play in collision and high-velocity sports after ACDF are healed arthrodesis at all levels, full functional range of motion of the cervical spine, and no residual neurologic deficit[19,28,36,37,41,47–50,53] (See Box 1). Assessment of final fusion should be based on radiographic or computed tomography imaging, with criteria from Rhee and colleagues[54] (Table 3). Fusion assessment on plain radiographs includes a lateral image with early bony bridging at the vertebral body interface, and lateral dynamic flexion and extension films that demonstrate less than 1 mm of motion between spinous processes. In addition, for athletes with findings of focal spinal stenosis on preoperative MRI, a postoperative MRI should be considered to confirm adequate decompression before returning to collision and high-velocity sports.[37] Furthermore, residual hyperintensity of the cord does not necessarily preclude participation as long as the source of neurocompression has been eliminated with restoration of canal dimmensions.[37,39] Overall, these recommendations are based on expert opinion and clinical experience of the authors, with limited evidence-based data.[37]

In addition to ACDF, there are several other possible surgical treatments for cervical disc herniation and spondylosis causing symptomatic stenosis, which include

---

Box 1
Return to play criteria after anterior cervical discectomy and fusion

- Solid arthrodesis at all levels.
- Full functional range of motion of the cervical spine.
- No residual neurologic deficit.
- Postoperative MRI should be considered to confirm adequate decompression if athlete with preoperative focal spinal stenosis.

Table 3
Radiographic criteria for evaluation of cervical fusion

Imaging Method	Criteria for Fusion
Plain radiograph	Static • Presence of bone trabeculation across the graft–host interface • Presence of bridging bone across the graft into the adjacent endplates, or bridging bone outside the graft and no lucent line (extending >50% of the graft-host bone interface) Dynamic • Interspinous process motion <1 mm, with assessment of superjacent interspinous motion with cutoff of ≤4 mm at 150% magnification • Cobb angle <2° on lateral flexion–extension • Presence of trabeculae bridging of the graft–vertebral body gap and absence of motion at the spinour process
Computed tomography	• Presence of bridging trabeculae across fusion level and graft • No lucent lines crossing peripheral margins and complete cortical bridging • Radiolucency at the graft vertebral junction
MRI	• Evidence of bony bridging from endplate to endplate without signal alteration at the graft–vertebral body junction

Adapted from Rhee JM, Chapman JR, Norvell DC, et al. Radiological determination of postoperative cervical fusion: a systematic review. Spine 2015;40:974–91.

posterior laminectomy and fusion, as well as nonfusion options such as cervical disc arthroplasty, posterior laminoforaminotomy, and posterior laminaplasty. To our knowledge, there is no available literature regarding these other treatment options and return to play in athletes, but the general criteria for return to play should apply including full functional cervical range of motion, with no residual neurologic deficits, or areas of neurocompression, and for posterior cervical fusion healed arthrodesis at all levels. Some authors have suggested that athletes may achieve a quicker recovery after nonfusion surgery, such as laminoforaminotomy, but a direct comparison

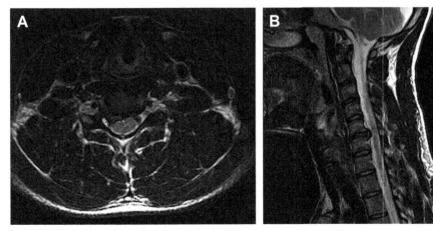

Fig. 1. (*A, B*) Axial and sagittal T2-weighted MRI of acute disc herniation causing radiculopathy in a 23-year-old male, National Collegiate Athletic Association Division 1 wrestler.

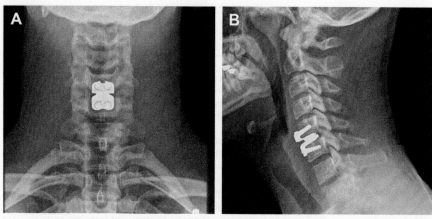

Fig. 2. (*A, B*) Postoperative anteroposterior and lateral radiographs of a 23-year-old male, National Collegiate Athletic Association Division 1 Wrestler at 1-year after single-level cervical disc arthroplasty. Athlete returned to play within 3 months after the operation and competed in a national championship tournament.

between the different types of surgery in athletes is unavailable.[15,52,55] However, even unilateral posterior laminoforamintomy with discectomy performed using minimal exposure has the potential to destabilize the operated segment; therefore, lateral dynamic flexion and extension films should be considered before return to play.[56] In addition, after posterior laminaplasty the complete healing of the hinge portion of the lamina must be considered. However, the duration of time for complete healing and restoration of the lamina strength to withstand high-energy loads remains unknown.[39] Although cervical disc arthroplasty seems to be a reasonable option given the risk of adjacent segment degeneration and disease after ACDF, the longevity of these devices with repetitive loading in collision athletes is unknown (**Figs. 1** and **2**). Also in patients with preoperative cord contusion, the fusion treatment option prevents hypermobility of the spinal segment and maintains the space available for the cord, whereas nonfusion treatment such as cervical disc arthroplasty or posterior laminaplasty may not provide protection from recurrent spinal canal impingement or hypermobility.[39]

SUMMARY

Decision making to allow a professional or elite athlete to return to play can be challenging for the surgeon, athlete, and their family and coaches. The possibility of a catastrophic SCI remains one of the major concerns for return to play after cervical disc surgery, although there has been no report of such an injury.[1,5,26,37] However, the available literature on outcomes and return to play criteria is limited, and the risk factors for catastrophic injury are not well-defined. In addition, the risk–benefit ratio can be aligned or completely diametric depending on the value system and biases of the athlete and surgeon.[19] Therefore, determining return to play criteria after surgery remains more of an art than a science, and continues to depend on the experience and good judgment of the treating surgeon, while taking into account the limited available guidelines.[52] There is strong consensus in the literature, despite lack of evidence based data, that athletes after single-level ACDF may safely return to play in collision and high-velocity sports. However, controversy remains for longer ACDF constructs and other fusion and nonfusion surgical treatment options. The athlete should be counseled and managed on a case-by-case basis, taking into consideration the type of sport, player specific variables (level of play, position, symptoms, history), and type of surgery performed.[6]

REFERENCES

1. Hsu WK. Outcomes following nonoperative and operative treatment for cervical disc herniations in National Football League athletes. Spine 2011;36:800–5.
2. Schroeder GD, Lynch TS, Gibbs DB, et al. The impact of a cervical spine diagnosis on the careers of National Football League athletes. Spine 2014;39:947–52.
3. Radhakrishnan K, Litchy WJ, O'Fallon WM, et al. Epidemiology of cervical radiculopathy. A population-based study from Rochester, Minnesota, 1976 through 1990. Brain 1994;117(Pt 2):325–35.
4. Vaccaro AR, Klein GR, Ciccoti M, et al. Return to play criteria for the athlete with cervical spine injuries resulting in stinger and transient quadriplegia/paresis. Spine J 2002;2:351–6.
5. Mall NA, Buchowski J, Zebala L, et al. Spine and axial skeleton injuries in the National Football League. Am J Sports Med 2012;40:1755–61.
6. Triantafillou KM, Lauerman W, Kalantar SB. Degenerative disease of the cervical spine and its relationship to athletes. Clin Sports Med 2012;31:509–20.
7. Hadler NM. Illness in the workplace: the challenge of musculoskeletal symptoms. J Hand Surg 1985;10:451–6.
8. Lawrence JS. Disc degeneration. Its frequency and relationship to symptoms. Ann Rheum Dis 1969;28:121–38.
9. Boden SD, McCowin PR, Davis DO, et al. Abnormal magnetic-resonance scans of the cervical spine in asymptomatic subjects. A prospective investigation. J Bone Joint Surg Am 1990;72:1178–84.
10. Gore DR, Sepic SB, Gardner GM. Roentgenographic findings of the cervical spine in asymptomatic people. Spine 1986;11:521–4.
11. Matsumoto M, Fujimura Y, Suzuki N, et al. MRI of cervical intervertebral discs in asymptomatic subjects. J Bone Joint Surg Am 1998;80:19–24.
12. Kelsey JL, Githens PB, Walter SD, et al. An epidemiological study of acute prolapsed cervical intervertebral disc. J Bone Joint Surg Am 1984;66:907–14.
13. Albright JP, Moses JM, Feldick HG, et al. Nonfatal cervical spine injuries in interscholastic football. JAMA 1976;236:1243–5.
14. Roberts DW, Roc GJ, Hsu WK. Outcomes of cervical and lumbar disk herniations in Major League Baseball pitchers. Orthopedics 2011;34:602–9.
15. Mundt DJ, Kelsey JL, Golden AL, et al. An epidemiologic study of sports and weight lifting as possible risk factors for herniated lumbar and cervical discs. The Northeast Collaborative Group on Low Back Pain. Am J Sports Med 1993; 21:854–60.
16. Jonasson P, Halldin K, Karlsson J, et al. Prevalence of joint-related pain in the extremities and spine in five groups of top athletes. Knee Surg Sports Traumatol Arthrosc 2011;19:1540–6.
17. Berge J, Marque B, Vital JM, et al. Age-related changes in the cervical spines of front-line rugby players. Am J Sports Med 1999;27:422–9.
18. Hogan BA, Hogan NA, Vos PM, et al. The cervical spine of professional front-row rugby players: correlation between degenerative changes and symptoms. Ir J Med Sci 2010;179:259–63.

19. Dailey A, Harrop JS, France JC. High-energy contact sports and cervical spine neuropraxia injuries: what are the criteria for return to participation? Spine 2010;35:S193–201.

20. Mehnert MJ, Agesen T, Malanga GA. "Heading" and neck injuries in soccer: a review of biomechanics and potential long-term effects. Pain Physician 2005;8: 391–7.

21. Tysvaer AT. Head and neck injuries in soccer. Impact of minor trauma. Sports Med 1992;14:200–13.

22. Tsirikos A, Papagelopoulos PJ, Giannakopoulos PN, et al. Degenerative spondyloarthropathy of the cervical and lumbar spine in jockeys. Orthopedics 2001;24: 561–4.

23. Weir DR, Jackson JS, Sonnega A. National football league player care foundation study of retired NFL players. Available at: http://ns.umich.edu/Releases/2009/Sep09/FinalReport.pdf. Accessed January 15, 2016.

24. Smith MG, Fulcher M, Shanklin J, et al. The prevalence of congenital cervical spinal stenosis in 262 college and high school football players. J Ky Med Assoc 1993;91:273–5.

25. Gray BL, Buchowski JM, Bumpass DB, et al. Disc herniations in the National Football League. Spine 2013;38:1934–8.

26. Meredith DS, Jones KJ, Barnes R, et al. Operative and nonoperative treatment of cervical disc herniation in National Football League athletes. Am J Sports Med 2013;41:2054–8.

27. Powell JW, Barber-Foss KD. Injury patterns in selected high school sports: a review of the 1995-1997 seasons. J Athl Train 1999;34:277–84.

28. Andrews J, Jones A, Davies PR, et al. Is return to professional rugby union likely after anterior cervical spinal surgery? J Bone Joint Surg Am 2008;90:619–21.

29. Scher AT. Premature onset of degenerative disease of the cervical spine in rugby players. S Afr Med J 1990;77:557–8.

30. Quarrie KL, Cantu RC, Chalmers DJ. Rugby union injuries to the cervical spine and spinal cord. Sports Med 2002;32:633–53.

31. Thomas BE, McCullen GM, Yuan HA. Cervical spine injuries in football players. J Am Acad Orthop Surg 1999;7:338–47.

32. Spinal Cord Injury Model Systems. NSCISC National Spinal Cord Injury Statistical Center. NSCISC Annual Statistical Report Complete Public Version.pdf. Available at: www.nscisc.uab.edu/PublicDocuments/reports/pdf/2014. Accessed January 15, 2016.

33. Tator CH, Edmonds VE, New ML. Diving: a frequent and potentially preventable cause of spinal cord injury. Can Med Assoc J 1981;124:1323–4.

34. Kepler CK, Vaccaro AR. Injuries and abnormalities of the cervical spine and return to play criteria. Clin Sports Med 2012;31:499–508.

35. Boden BP, Tacchetti RL, Cantu RC, et al. Catastrophic cervical spine injuries in high school and college football players. Am J Sports Med 2006;34:1223–32.

36. Tator CH, Provvidenza C, Cassidy JD. Update and Overview of Spinal Injuries in Canadian Ice Hockey, 1943 to 2011: The Continuing Need for Injury Prevention and Education. Clin J Sport Med 2016;26(3):232–8.

37. Maroon JC, Bost JW, Petraglia AL, et al. Outcomes after anterior cervical discectomy and fusion in professional athletes. Neurosurgery 2013;73:103–12 [discussion: 12].

38. Maroon JC, El-Kadi H, Abla AA, et al. Cervical neurapraxia in elite athletes: evaluation and surgical treatment. Report of five cases. J Neurosurg Spine 2007;6: 356–63.

39. Brigham CD, Capo J. Cervical spinal cord contusion in professional athletes: a case series with implications for return to play. Spine 2013;38:315–23.
40. Saigal R, Batjer HH, Ellenbogen RG, et al. Return to play for neurosurgical patients. World Neurosurg 2014;82:485–91.
41. Jeyamohan S, Harrop JS, Vaccaro A, et al. Athletes returning to play after cervical spine or neurobrachial injury. Curr Rev Musculoskelet Med 2008;1:175–9.
42. Morganti C, Sweeney CA, Albanese SA, et al. Return to play after cervical spine injury. Spine 2001;26:1131–6.
43. Cantu RC, Mueller FO. Catastrophic spine injuries in football (1977-1989). J Spinal Disord 1990;3:227–31.
44. Torg JS. Epidemiology, pathomechanics, and prevention of athletic injuries to the cervical spine. Med Sci Sports Exerc 1985;17:295–303.
45. Wadley GH, Albright JP. Women's intercollegiate gymnastics. Injury patterns and "permanent" medical disability. Am J Sports Med 1993;21:314–20.
46. Kiely P, Baker JF, O'HEireamhoin S, et al. The evaluation of the inverted supinator reflex in asymptomatic patients. Spine 2010;35:955–7.
47. Torg JS, Ramsey-Emrhein JA. Suggested management guidelines for participation in collision activities with congenital, developmental, or postinjury lesions involving the cervical spine. Med Sci Sports Exerc 1997;29:S256–72.
48. Burnett MG, Sonntag VK. Return to contact sports after spinal surgery. Neurosurg Focus 2006;21:E5.
49. Morganti C. Recommendations for return to sports following cervical spine injuries. Sports Med 2003;33:563–73.
50. Vaccaro AR, Watkins B, Albert TJ, et al. Cervical spine injuries in athletes: current return-to-play criteria. Orthopedics 2001;24:699–703 [quiz: 4–5].
51. Torg JS, Ramsey-Emrhein JA. Management guidelines for participation in collision activities with congenital, developmental, or post-injury lesions involving the cervical spine. Clin Sports Med 1997;16:501–30.
52. Zmurko MG, Tannoury TY, Tannoury CA, et al. Cervical sprains, disc herniations, minor fractures, and other cervical injuries in the athlete. Clin Sports Med 2003;22:513–21.
53. Torg JS. Cervical spine injuries and the return to football. Sports Health 2009;1:376–83.
54. Rhee JM, Chapman JR, Norvell DC, et al. Radiological Determination of Postoperative Cervical Fusion: A Systematic Review. Spine 2015;40:974–91.
55. Tumialan LM, Ponton RP, Gluf WM. Management of unilateral cervical radiculopathy in the military: the cost effectiveness of posterior cervical foraminotomy compared with anterior cervical discectomy and fusion. Neurosurg Focus 2010;28:E17.
56. Micheli LJ. Sports following spinal surgery in the young athlete. Clin Orthop Relat Res 1985;(198):152–7.

Return to Play Following Anterior Shoulder Dislocation and Stabilization Surgery

Michael A. Donohue, MD[a], Brett D. Owens, MD[b],
Jonathan F. Dickens, MD[a],*

KEYWORDS

- Shoulder • Dislocation • Subluxation • Instability • Return to play • Sports
- Bankart

KEY POINTS

- Athletes, especially contact, collision, and overhead athletes, are an at-risk population for anterior glenohumeral instability and their treatment depends on a variety of factors, including acuity, time in season, and long-term career goals.
- In-season athletes may be initially treated nonoperatively with an accelerated rehabilitation protocol if they meet specific criteria to complete their season. Nonoperative treatment, however, has a high rate of recurrence despite return to play.
- Arthroscopic and open Bankart repair are both reliable treatment options with a trend towards decreased recurrence using open Bankart repair for contact and collision athletes.
- Open osseous augmentation procedures should be used for athletes with greater than 20% to 25% glenoid bone loss.

INTRODUCTION

The shoulder represents the most mobile joint in the body of the athlete, providing the greatest arc of motion across multiple planes with a combination of static and dynamic stabilizers necessary for maintenance of joint congruity. However, with such range of

Funding: None.
Conflicts of Interest: None (M.A. Donohue and J.F. Dickens); Pacira pharmaceuticals (Shareholder); consultant for Mitek and MTF/Conmed Linvatec (B.D. Owens).
Disclaimer: The views expressed in this presentation are those of the authors and do not necessarily reflect the official policy or position of the Department of the Army, the Defense Health Agency, the Department of Defense, or the US government.
[a] Department of Orthopaedic Surgery, Walter Reed National Military Medical Center, Building 19, Floor 2, 8901 Wisconsin Avenue, Bethesda, MD 20889, USA; [b] Department of Orthopaedics, Brown Alpert Medical School, 100 Butler Drive, Providence, RI 02906, USA
* Corresponding author.
E-mail address: jonathan.f.dickens.mil@mail.mil

motion, the osseous architecture is relatively unconstrained and shallow, allowing both translation and rotation, thus leaving the glenohumeral joint at risk for dislocation.[1] Glenohumeral joint instability, including both dislocation and subluxation, accounts for the most common joint instability (17 per 10,000 per year) and very commonly occurs in young, especially male, athletes.[2,3] Most of these events are anterior inferior subluxations or dislocations. Management of athletes and returning them to play in an expeditious but safe manner includes both nonoperative and operative modalities based on thorough discussion of expectations, limitations, level of play, and time left in season.[4,5] The authors briefly review the anatomy and pathologic condition of anterior shoulder instability, and the workup and diagnosis of anterior shoulder instability in the athlete. Finally, the authors review return to play (RTP) outcomes for these athletes given the various treatment options: nonoperative, arthroscopic repair, open repair, and open osseous augmentation.

Anatomy

The glenohumeral articulation relies on both the osseous structure and soft tissues surrounding the shoulder for static and dynamic restraint. The relatively convex pear-shaped glenoid and spherical humeral head articulate similar to a golf ball on tee, affording stability through concavity compression generated through surrounding soft tissues and negative joint pressure.[6,7] In addition to the concave nature of the glenoid, the labrum provides increased depth in static stabilization of the humeral head.[8] The glenohumeral ligaments are important static stabilizers and provide restraint throughout the arc of motion (**Table 1**). The anterior band of inferior glenohumeral ligament is the primary static restraint to anterior translation of the abducted and externally rotated arm.[6,8] Dynamic stabilizers include the rotator cuff, long head of the biceps, deltoid, and muscles of the scapula.

Pathoanatomy

Traumatic anterior dislocation can injure both bone and soft tissue restraints. The Bankart lesion (avulsion of the anterior inferior glenoid labrum), described in 1923,[9] has been shown by Arciero and Taylor[10] to have an incidence as high as 97% in collegiate athletes with a 90% incidence of Hill-Sachs lesions. Biomechanical testing with a sectioned labrum leads to decreased force to cause dislocation by up to 20%.[11] Similarly, a first-time traumatic anterior subluxation event has been shown to result in high rates of Bankart lesions (96%), described by Owens and colleagues.[12] Whether acute or repetitive in nature, anterior shoulder dislocation may also lead attritional bone loss with multiple recurrences.[10,13,14] Bone loss greater than 20% to 25% risks continued instability with arthroscopic stabilization techniques and has been traditionally considered an indication for open stabilization with bone augmentation. Biomechanical testing of this critical limit of bone loss has shown a significant destabilization of the glenohumeral joint and risks continued instability. In contact athletes,

Table 1 Glenohumeral ligament functions		
Ligament	**Arm Position**	**Prevents Translation**
Superior	Adducted	Anterior or inferior
Middle	45° abducted	Anterior or inferior
Anterior-inferior band	90° abducted or external rotation	Anterior
Posterior-inferior band	90° abducted or internal rotation	Posterior

bone loss between 10% and 20% may also be a risk factor for recurrence.[15–17] Other associated lesions that may occur include the anterior labral periosteal sleeve avulsion, humeral avulsion of the glenohumeral ligament (HAGL), and glenolabral articular disruption.

Incidence

Shoulder instability in the athlete can lead to disability as well as significant time lost to sports. In 2009, Owens and colleagues[3] published a National Collegiate Athletic Association (NCAA) Injury Surveillance System data analysis of 4080 glenohumeral instability events in college athletes and reported a rate of 0.12 per 1000 exposures, most of which were contact events, with the highest occurrences in wrestling, football, and ice hockey. Almost half of these events required at least 10 days out of sport for the injured player. Among US high school students, football and wrestling represent the highest incidence of shoulder instability. In rugby players, most dislocations occur in direct contact with other players and represent a mean of 81 days lost to sport.[18] Whereas most epidemiologic study of shoulder instability has focused on dislocation events, 1 study of a collegiate-aged population showed that subluxation events compose 85% of all instability events.[19] Clearly, shoulder instability in the athlete is a significant source of injury and time lost from sport.

PATIENT EVALUATION
History

The acuity of presentation of an athlete with shoulder instability ranges a full spectrum from sideline, training room, and clinic. Essential for diagnosis is a complete and thorough history and physical examination The initial history gathering can come from the injured athlete; on-field staff; athletic trainers; and, if available, recorded video of specific events demonstrating contact versus noncontact event and the mechanism of injury.[20] Athletes who sustain a single acute traumatic event may recall the exact timing of the inciting trauma and mechanism of the injury, although those who have sustained multiple instability events, especially those who only have subluxations, may have nonspecific recollection of initial injury as well as incomplete recall of total number of events.[12,19]

A thorough patient history should begin with determination of patient age at the initial event as well as chronologic timing of any subsequent events, because age at initial injury has prognostic value for recurrence of instability.[21–23] The type and mechanism of injury, as well as position of the arm at time of injury, can provide important diagnostic clues regarding the injury pattern and may also describe multidirectional instability or generalized laxity. Associated symptoms, including neurologic deficits,[24] and determination of chronology of other interventions, whether rest, physical therapy, or other, enhance the surgeon's understanding of the patient's current pathologic condition.

The patient's sports played (contact vs noncontact, **Table 2**), level of play, current time into season, and patient expectation to continue at current level of play or career plans are essential factors for the surgeon to consider and helps to guide medical decision-making. Especially in the setting of low-energy injuries or multiple bilateral events, the patient's past medical history can provide insight to potential connective tissue disorders, whether diagnosed or undiagnosed, and includes documentation of instability in any other joints as well as treatments received.

Physical Examination

The physical examination of the athlete's shoulder is critical to aid in decision-making for returning an athlete to play in-season versus recommending surgical stabilization. A

Table 2
Classification of sports as contact or collision, limited contact, and noncontact from the American Academy of Pediatrics

Contact or Collision	Limited Contact	Noncontact
Basketball	Baseball	Archery
Boxing[a]	Bicycling	Badminton
Diving	Cheerleading	Body building
Field hockey	Canoeing or kayaking (white water)	Bowling
Football	Fencing	Canoeing or kayaking (flat water)
Flag	Field	Crew or rowing
Tackle	High jump	Curling
Ice hockey	Pole vault	Dancing
Lacrosse	Floor hockey	Field
Martial arts	Gymnastics	Discus
Rodeo	Handball	Javelin
Rugby	Horseback riding	Shot put
Ski jumping	Racquetball	Golf
Soccer	Skating	Orienteering
Team handball	Ice	Power lifting
Water polo	Inline	Race walking
Wrestling	Roller	Riflery
	Skiing	Rope jumping
	Cross-country	Running
	Downhill	Sailing
	Water	Scuba diving
	Softball	Strength training
	Squash	Swimming
	Ultimate Frisbee	Table tennis
	Volleyball	Tennis
	Windsurfing or surfing	Track
		Weight lifting

[a] Indicates sport not recommended for young athletes.

(*Adapted from* Rice SG. Medical conditions affecting sports participation. American Academy of Pediatrics Committee on Sports Medicine and Fitness. Pediatrics 1994;94(5):757–60.)

complete physical examination includes examination of the injured and uninjured shoulders' skin, muscles, distal innervations, and all motions of the humerus and scapula. See later discussion of specific provocative examinations to elucidate shoulder instability.

Apprehension test or relocation test

The apprehension test has been described as a highly specific test for predicting recurrent instability and is among the most common positive findings.[25,26] The maneuver is performed with the humerus abducted to 90° and externally rotated. An anteriorly directed force is applied to the shoulder and the test is considered positive only if there is apprehension or guarding. In the absence of apprehension or guarding, a finding of pain alone may suggest subtle instability.[4,26] In 1989, Jobe and colleagues[27] described an addition to this test commonly referred to as the relocation test. In the supine patient, with the arm in the apprehensive position, the examiner places a posteriorly directed force to the anterior shoulder. A positive relocation test will relieve the patient of apprehension and guarding. The most sensitive maneuver to complete this provocative test is the surprise test, according to pooled data from a 2012 meta-analysis.[28] In the surprise test, the examiner completes relocation and then suddenly releases the posteriorly directed force. When this occurs, the patient will again feel a sudden onset of apprehension or instability.

Load and shift test

The load and shift test is a graded provocative examination on a scale from 1 through 3 indicating the degree of translation of the humeral head. An axial load is applied to the shoulder through the humerus at the elbow, which centers the humeral head in the glenoid fossa; then anterior and posterior directed force is applied to the humeral head with the examiner's other hand. The test is performed incrementally from an adducted shoulder at 0° to 90° of shoulder abduction. Grade I represents increased translation compared with the contralateral side or normal shoulder. Grade II represents translation to the glenoid rim. Grade III represents the ability to translate the humeral head over the glenoid rim or even to frankly dislocate the shoulder.[4] The efficacy of the load and shift test has been questioned and found to be poorly sensitive but highly specific with range of specificity from 89.9% to 98%.[29,30]

Other provocative maneuvers

Evaluation of multidirectional instability as well as generalized ligamentous laxity should also be performed. Posterior instability can be tested with the use of the posterior load and shift, the Kim test, and the Jerk test. Ligamentous laxity may be evaluated using the Beighton hypermobility score. Additionally, evaluation of laxity specific to anterior instability is done using the Gagey test. The Gagey test examines inferior glenohumeral ligament laxity if the arm can be abducted beyond 105° without scapular motion. The Gagey test and external rotation of the adducted arm greater than 90° have been shown by Boileau and colleagues[31] to represent risk factors for recurrent postoperative instability (**Table 3**).

Imaging

Imaging provides the diagnostic insight of an athlete's pathologic condition and helps determine if an athlete may be able to be released to play in the same season with nonoperative treatment. Initial plain films are required to verify a reduced glenohumeral joint, and may provide additional evaluation of the inferior glenoid in the case of a bony Bankart or loss of contour, as well as the humeral head for Hill-Sachs lesions. Initial imaging series of shoulder include true anterior-posterior (AP) of the glenohumeral joint, axillary lateral, and scapular Y. The AP view of the shoulder may be obtained with humeral internal or external rotation, although some investigators have advocated

Table 3 Essential portions of the patient encounter	
History	**Physical Examination**
• Age and timing at most recent instability event • Mechanism of injury as well as position of arm at time of injury • Acute vs recurrent or chronic (chronicle number of events) • Subluxation vs dislocation • Sport played (contact vs noncontact) and time left in season; also must determine goals for continued sports career • Other similar events in other joints and previous surgical interventions	• General inspection and palpation for any gross abnormalities • Range of motion in multiple planes: forward flexion, abduction, external rotation, internal rotation • Strength and neurologic testing: rotator cuff, deltoid, axillary nerve, distal innervations • Special tests: sulcus sign, Apprehension or relocation test; Load & shift test (anterior and posterior), jerk test, Gagey test • Laxity: Beighton score: elbow (2), thumb (2), finger (2), knee (2), trunk forward flexion (1) • Thorough examination of contralateral shoulder

for the use of the external rotation AP.[32] Other views providing high-yield evaluation of the osseous contours are the West Point view to assess the glenoid and the Stryker Notch to evaluate the Hill-Sachs lesion.[33] A bony Bankart seen on plain films precludes an athlete from same-season RTP.

MRI and MR angiography (MRA) allow evaluation in multiple 2-dimensional planes, as well as reconstructed 3-dimensional planes. Acutely traumatized athletes with anterior shoulder dislocations develop capsular distention from hemarthrosis, which enhances visualization of the soft tissue interfaces throughout the joint that are pathognomonic of anterior shoulder instability, namely the Bankart lesion, Perthes lesion, anterior labral periosteal sleeve avulsion, and HAGL.[34,35] In the subacute and chronic setting, infiltration and distention of the glenohumeral joint is achieved with gadolinium contrast dye.

In addition to soft-tissue imaging, MRI and MRA allow visualization of the osseous architecture of the glenoid and humeral head, as well as resulting edema underlying cortical bone from acute trauma. As originally described, the Hill-Sachs lesion is a posteriorly based humeral head compression resultant from traumatic dislocation.[36] MRI or MRA imaging can demonstrate edema in the posterior humeral head in the absence of frank bone loss.[12] Recently, the concept of the glenoid track and calculation of humeral bone loss for predicting engaging Hill-Sachs lesions has been investigated and will be discussed in the section on computed tomography (CT) imaging.[37]

In an effort to reduce patient exposure to radiation, as well a limit the amount of advanced imaging studies the patient undergoes, methods to calculate glenoid bone loss have been introduced using MRI or MRA. Owens and colleagues[38] prospectively followed US Military Academy cadets and obtained bilateral shoulder MRIs of young athletes. After review of greater than 1200 shoulder MRIs, a significant relationship between glenoid height (H) and width (W) in millimeters was found. The researchers developed a formula to predict expected normal glenoid width: male patients: $W = (1/3\,H) + 15$ mm; female patients: $W = (1/3\,H) + 13$ mm. Using this simple calculation of expected glenoid width, glenoid bone loss can be estimated by comparing the value to actual glenoid width.

Using ionizing radiation, CT imaging offers rapid acquisition multiplanar imaging most beneficial for assessing bone loss. Although introduction of arthrogram contrast dye may improve soft tissue visualization, CT is often reserved for suspected glenoid bone loss, bony Bankart lesions, large Hill-Sachs lesions, failed previous repairs, and patients with a contraindication to MRI or MRA.[4,34]

Humeral bone loss in the Hill-Sachs lesion, though described in 1940, has regained awareness since a landmark study by Burkhart and DeBeer[16] identified that two-thirds of their failed Bankart repair patients had significant bone loss represented by either an engaging Hill-Sachs lesion or inverted-pear glenoid. Since this time, several methods using best-fit circles and edge-edge measurements have been developed to calculate humeral bone loss and likelihood of engagement.

Multiple techniques have been described for quantification of glenoid bone loss and use either a linear method or surface-area method of calculation of bone loss. Recently, Bhatia and colleagues,[39] have called into question the linear-based glenoid width method for overestimating actual bone loss. In general, bone loss greater than 20% to 25% is considered critical bone loss and portends a significant risk of recurrent instability in the absence of bony augmentation procedures.[16,31,32,40]

Treatment Options

Traumatic anterior shoulder instability leads to a significant amount of time lost from sport and may preclude participation in competitive sports for the remainder of the season. Whether the athlete wishes to RTP rapidly and pursues initial nonoperative management to complete the season, or elects to terminate play for the season and undergo surgical stabilization, the surgeon's goal is to expeditiously but safely return the athlete to play at similar levels from recreational to elite while preventing recurrent injury. Decision-making for each athlete is unique and depends on a variety of factors, including age, level of play, chronicity, and risk of recurrence, and career goals.

Nonoperative

In a prospective observational cohort study among NCAA college athletes, the US Military Academy, US Naval Academy, and US Air Force Academy examined in-season RTP following anterior shoulder instability events (dislocation or subluxation) over a 2-year period and found that 73% of intercollegiate athletes were able to return to complete all or part of their season with a mean of less than 1 week of time missed from competition. More concerning however, only 27% were able to successfully complete their season without recurrence of instability.[5] In a previous review, the same investigators suggested an algorithm for management of in-season athletes and contraindications for RTP following nonoperative treatment.[4] Contraindications include failure of nonoperative treatment, large and engaging Hill-Sachs lesions, glenoid bone loss greater than 20%, previous failed stabilization procedure, and HAGL lesions (**Fig. 1**).

RTP following traumatic anterior shoulder instability represents a spectrum of diagnoses, both acute and chronic in nature. In the right setting, RTP in the same season may be feasible but the athlete, athletic trainer, coach, and other members involved in the patient's care need to be in agreement. The greatest risk to a player is returning them to sport before it is safe to do so and risking further injury to the shoulder. Additionally, complications related to surgical procedures are not benign and must be balanced with the need for a stable glenohumeral joint based on multiple patient factors.

After initial reduction, nonsurgical management of the athlete involves a variety of treatment options that have been debated throughout the literature and can be broken into 3 main categories: (1) immobilization, (2) physical therapy, and (3) bracing.

Immobilization

After reduction, the arm is traditionally placed in a sling with the arm adducted and internally rotated for comfort of the patient. After a brief period of immobilization, athletes begin motion exercises, strengthening, and functional activities under the supervision of physical therapists or athletic trainers. In the course of transitioning out of sling and back to normal activities, some have questioned both the utility and the duration of immobilization, as well as the most appropriate position for immobilized arm.

One of the earliest challenges to sling use was by Hovelius and colleagues.[41] They prospectively followed 2 groups of subjects treated for initial anterior shoulder dislocation. One group was immobilized with slings for 3 to 4 weeks, while the second group was not immobilized and was encouraged to begin early motion and use of the shoulder. At 2-year follow-up, there was no difference in recurrence rate but, interestingly, subjects younger than 22 years old had nearly 50% recurrence. In their multicenter military academies study, Dickens and colleagues[5] did not use immobilization and emphasized an accelerated rehabilitation program,[4] returning 73% of players to their sport at a median of 5 days. The other 27% failed to regain shoulder function and underwent early elective surgery. One other study also evaluated in-season athletes and immobilization but retrospectively. Buss and colleagues[42] reviewed 30 shoulder instability events in young athletes. No subjects were immobilized and all underwent physical therapy. In these athletes, a mean of 10.2 days were lost with 90% returning to same level of play but with a 37% recurrence rate. The timeline of missed

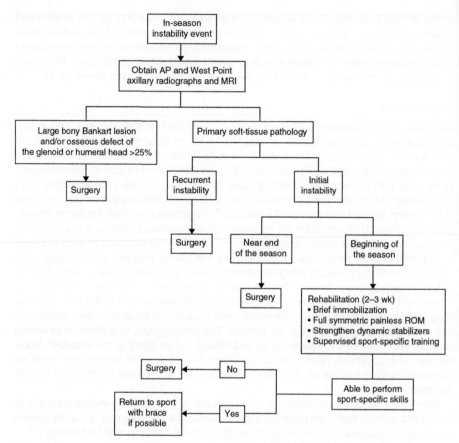

Fig. 1. RTP and surgical decision-making algorithm. ROM, range of motion. (*From* Owens BD, Dickens JF, Kilcoyne KG, et al. Management of mid-season traumatic anterior shoulder instability in athletes. J Am Acad Orthop Surg 2012;20(8):518–26.)

sport days is heterogeneous among the 2 papers, with 1 reporting a mean and the other median; however, both reported relatively few days missed and high percentage (pooled = 80%) RTP in the same season.

Also debated in sling use following anterior shoulder instability is the positioning of the arm, which may affect displacement of the anterior labrum. Itoi and colleagues[40] initially presented MRI findings of improved reduction of Bankart lesions with the arm in approximately 35° of external rotation. This was followed by a nonrandomized and a subsequent randomized trial that demonstrated a significant risk reduction in recurrence.[43,44] Other investigators have attempted to repeat these findings with less success. A systematic review and meta-analysis of level I and II studies failed to find any significant difference in rotation of the arm and its effects on recurrent instability.[45] With the variety of outcomes reported, the investigators recommended judicious use of a sling for only a brief time for in-season athletes who meet potential RTP criteria in the same season.

Physical therapy

To return athletes to play during the same season, physical therapy can facilitate achievement of baseline goals, including minimal pain, symmetric motion and strength, and functional performance with specific exercises.[4,5,20,46] Many supervised physical therapy programs exist and have similar progression back to sport. The authors recommend early range of motion, followed by stabilization and strengthening, and return to sport once the previously discussed criteria is met.

Brace wear

To date, no study exists demonstrating reduced shoulder instability rates with use of a motion-limiting brace; yet, for many athletes, brace wear is recommended.[20] Caution should be exercised with throwing or overhead athletes who rely on abduction and external rotation, especially in their dominant arm, because the brace will inherently limit these motions.

Nonoperative management of anterior shoulder instability in the athlete relies on early diagnosis and an initial period of rest, followed by streamlined return to phased rehabilitation protocol. In the setting of chronic instability, continued nonoperative management should not be recommended.

Surgical Treatment Algorithm

Following the acute anterior shoulder dislocation, the young athlete may elect to undergo surgical stabilization due to continued and recurrent instability, preventing full return to sport or participation in an overhead, contact, or collision sports that requires a stable shoulder.[47] **Fig. 1** outlines the authors' recommended treatment algorithm. In-season athletes who elect to undergo operative management of anterior shoulder instability will not return to their sport in the current season because of time necessary for proper rehabilitation. Several criteria systems have been established to determine the optimal technique (arthroscopic repair, open repair, bone augmentation) to prevent recurrent instability. Essential to this decision is evaluation of glenoid bone loss. Additionally, when considering arthroscopic versus open surgical approaches, Balg and Boileau[32] have developed a 10-point instability severity index score (ISIS) (**Table 4**). Athletes who scored greater than 6 are at very high (~70%) risk for recurrent instability following arthroscopic repair.

Arthroscopic repair

Articles by Arciero and colleagues[21] and Wheeler and colleagues[48] described nonoperative versus arthroscopic treatment of acute first-time anterior shoulder dislocators and found a 80% to 92% rate of recurrent instability in those treated nonoperatively, whereas those treated with arthroscopic repair had a 12% to 14% rate of recurrent instability with 15 to 32 months of follow-up. With advances in modern arthroscopic techniques, a trend towards increasing use of arthroscopic Bankart repair has occurred (**Fig. 2**). However, some investigators have begun to question its utility, especially in contact and collision athletes. Mazzocca and colleagues[49] reported 37-month follow-ups on 18 contact or collision athletes, and reported an 11% recurrent dislocation rate, which is at least triple the rates reported in open subjects. All of the subjects returned to their previous level of play.

Gerometta and colleagues[50] published their results of 46 athletes with a mean of 2-year follow-up, as well as a literature review evaluating reported RTP rates of athletes. In their population, 95% returned to their sports but only 80% returned to their preinjury level. The recurrence rate was 2.4%. Athletes who sustained more than 10 dislocations preoperatively returned to sports at a significantly prolonged postoperative period compared with those with either less than 5 dislocations or a single dislocation event.

At the time of this article, there are 9 peer-reviewed articles that address recurrence and RTP following arthroscopic shoulder stabilization in contact and collision

Table 4 Instability severity index score scoring	
Prognostic Factors	**Points**
Age at surgery (y)	
≤20	2
>20	0
Degree of sport participation (preoperative)	
Competitive	2
Recreational or none	0
Type of sport (preoperative)	
Contact or forced overhead	1
Other	0
Shoulder hyperlaxity	
Anterior or inferior	1
Normal laxity	0
Hill-Sachs on AP radiograph	
Visible in external rotation	2
Not visible in external rotation	0
Glenoid loss of contour on AP radiograph	
Loss of contour	2
No lesion	0
Total (points)	10

From Balg F, Boileau P. The instability severity index score. A simple pre-operative score to select patients for arthroscopic or open shoulder stabilisation. J Bone Joint Surg Br 2007;89(11):1470–7; with permission.

athletes.[49,51–59] In the cumulative 361 young and predominantly male athletes, 73% RTP at their previous level of competition at a mean of 29 weeks postoperatively. After a mean follow-up period of 55 weeks, the recurrence rate was 14.2.[49,52–59]

Open repair
Despite improvement in recurrent instability rates, specific focus on contact athlete instability recurrence led to increasing concern that arthroscopic anterior shoulder

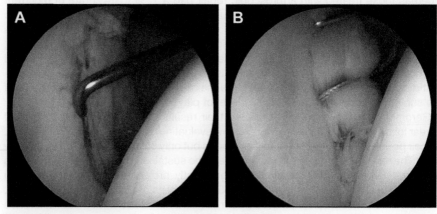

Fig. 2. (*A*) Arthroscopic view of a Bankart lesion and (*B*) completed repair.

stabilization may be insufficient.[56,60] When evaluating failure of open stabilization, multiple studies have reported recurrence rates in throwing athletes, contact athletes, and noncontact athletes, although not every study has delineated within their results the individual subgroup failure rates. Jobe and colleagues[61] reported zero recurrence in elite overhead athletes at a mean of 38 months follow-up. However, these results have not been similarly reported. Uhorchak and colleagues[62] evaluated 66 cadets at West Point with a mean of 47 months follow-up and reported a recurrence rate of 23%; however, only 3% of those were frank dislocation events that occurred during collision sports. The investigators reported that they had treated a variety of contact and overhead athletes. Bigliani and colleagues[63] also treated a variety of contact and overhead athletes, and reported a 2.9% recurrent dislocation rate but were unable to determine subluxation rates. The results suggest a very low redislocation rate underlying failure in athletes once they return to sports; however, shoulder subluxation may continue to be problematic for almost one-fourth of patients.

Recurrent instability and ability to return to sport vary based on the sport played and sport-specific requirements of the athlete. Jobe and colleagues[61] reported that only 72% of pitchers could return to preinjury level of play. In their subgroup analysis of overhead athletes, Bigliani and colleagues[63] found only 50% could return to the same level play, and even fewer (33%) professional or varsity level overheard players. Despite the 22% recurrence rate, Uhorchak and colleagues[62] reported that 100% returned their sports and completed military training.

In 2002, Pagnani and Dome[64] published 3-year follow-up results of open treatment of 58 American football players with recurrent instability. They reported a 0% dislocation rate postoperatively, with 89% of players returning to play for at least 1 more year. The authors reviewed the literature of RTP following anterior instability specifically in contact athletes. There are 6 publications, with 251 contact athletes treated with open stabilization without bone block augmentation. The recurrence rate was 13.6% with 76.9% returning to the previous level of play at an average of 26.1 weeks postoperatively.[58,59,62,64–66]

In 2014, Stone and Pearsall[67] conducted a systematic review of RTP criteria for athletes undergoing open Bankart repair. This study evaluated 29 articles published through 2012 and sought to determine specific timetable recommendations, as well as objective criteria, for RTP. The investigators were unable to find consistent objective criteria for release to sports; however, they do provide insight regarding timeline for return in athletes, as well as evaluation of recurrence rates. Noncontact athletes were released at 12 to 16 months postoperatively; whereas contact and throwing athletes returned to sports at 24 weeks. Twenty-one of the 29 articles provided redislocation rates with a mean of 5.3% (range 0%–11%). The minimum follow-up period for inclusion, however, was 8 months. Despite the in-depth review of timeline for return to sport, the study was lacking in a report of percentage of athletes who remained at the same level of play, moved to a lower level, or left sports all together.

Open osseous augmentation

For patients with significant glenoid bone loss of greater than 20% to 25%, an open bony augmentation is recommended. In the setting of a young contact athlete with shoulder instability, many of the ISIS scoring system risk factors are met and these athletes are high risk for recurrence postoperatively, regardless of quantified bone loss amount on CT scan or MRI. Walch and colleagues[68] retrospectively assessed 34 European rugby players (representing 37 shoulder stabilizations) who underwent a Latarjet procedure for recurrent anterior instability. Bone loss was not quantified. At an average of 12 years follow-up, no instability events occurred; however, 14% exhibited a positive apprehension test. All players were able to return to their previous level of play, with professional rugby players returning on average at 4 months to competition, whereas nonprofessional players returned to competition at 10 months postoperatively. Separately, 15-year follow-up data from Hovelius[69] report that out of 46 contact athletes treated with a Latarjet procedure, 3 (6.5%) left sports altogether and 2 (4.3%) had to lower their activity level. Unfortunately, the investigators did not distinguish any further characteristic of the athletes. There is insufficient and hetero-geneous data to attempt pooling of results in the Latarjet group regarding RTP.

Comparative outcomes

Few studies have provided a comparative evaluation of outcomes and RTP in the high-demand athlete population. Dickens and colleagues[70] prospectively evaluated the ability of contact and collision athletes to RTP with either nonoperative or arthro-scopic treatment. Thirty-nine contact athletes were eligible to play the season following surgical stabilization or nonoperative treatment. Of those, 10 athletes elec-ted nonoperative treatment, whereas 29 elected arthroscopic stabilization. The nonoperative group only achieved a 40% RTP rate, whereas the arthroscopic group achieved a 90% RTP rate without recurrent instability.

With a vast array of literature available regarding open and arthroscopic Bankart repair, and a moderate amount of literature regarding Latarjet procedures, several inves-tigators have attempted to conglomerate outcomes in systematic reviews. Harris and colleagues[71] evaluated 26 mostly level III and level IV studies with a mean follow-up of 11 years in more than 1700 subjects. This group was not specifically athletes but repre-sented the largest pooled subject data regarding open versus arthroscopic Bankart repairs. There was no significant difference in recurrent instability, 8% versus 11%, respectively. In studies that reported return to sports, there was a significant improve-ment in return to sport for those treated with open Bankart repair procedures, 89% versus 74% treated arthroscopically. However, subgroup analysis of arthroscopic su-ture anchor group versus open repair showed no significant difference in return to sports.

Most recently, Trantalis and colleagues[72] conducted a systematic review and meta-analysis of combined open or arthroscopic Bankart repair compared with Latarjet. Among their 8 included publications, there were 416 Bankart repairs and 379 open Latarjet procedures in a mostly male population. The mean age in both groups was 26 years old. Only half of the included studies, however, reported recurrence rate as an outcome. There was a significant 2-fold higher risk of recurrence for those treated with either open or arthroscopic Bankart compared with Latarjet. Open Bank-art repair demonstrated a trend to decreased recurrence compared with arthroscopic. All episodes of recurrence were subluxation events and no groups had any disloca-tions. There was no significant difference in the rates of revision surgery. Finally, RTP rates were all similar and not significantly different.

With increased rates of recurrent instability following nonoperative treatment of anterior glenohumeral instability, arthroscopic or open stabilization is generally per-formed. Despite a variety of literature indicating similar outcomes in RTP for operative management of anterior shoulder instability, there is a trend for decreased recurrence following open procedures versus arthroscopic. The meta-analysis presented previ-ously did not demonstrate a difference in RTP among athletes treated with Bankart repair or Latarjet. Further randomized trials and long-term follow-up specifically focused on the athlete subgroups needs to be conducted.

SUMMARY

The shoulder provides the greatest range of motion in multiple of all joints in the body but in conjunction with this comes decreased osseous constraint and increased risk for dislocation. The athlete, especially young collision and contact athletes, who sustain an anterior shoulder instability event, are at risk for continued instability without proper management. Allowing RTP in the same season is possible with the correct rehabilitation and may be done fairly expeditiously to reduce time lost from sports. However, careful evaluation of the patient's injury history, sports participation, physical examination, and radiologic findings are required. Arthroscopic and open anterior shoulder stabilization provide similar RTP for athletes, with significant differences in recurrence yet to be determined. However, any patient with critical bone loss greater than 20% to 25% should undergo open bone augmentation procedures to prevent future instability and, based on current literature, may still enjoy a high rate of return to previous level of play.

REFERENCES

1. Ghodadra N, Gupta A, Romeo AA, et al. Normalization of glenohumeral articular contact pressures after Latarjet or iliac crest bone-grafting. J Bone Joint Surg Am 2010;92(6):1478–89.

2. Kroner K, Lind T, Jensen J. The epidemiology of shoulder dislocations. Arch Orthop Trauma Surg 1989;108(5):288–90.

3. Owens BD, Agel J, Mountcastle SB, et al. Incidence of glenohumeral instability in collegiate athletics. Am J Sports Med 2009;37(9):1750–4.

4. Owens BD, Dickens JF, Kilcoyne KG, et al. Management of mid-season traumatic anterior shoulder instability in athletes. J Am Acad Orthop Surg 2012;20(8): 518–26.

5. Dickens JF, Owens BD, Cameron KL, et al. Return to play and recurrent instability after in-season anterior shoulder instability: a prospective multicenter study. Am J Sports Med 2014;42(12):2842–50.

6. Lippitt S, Matsen F. Mechanisms of glenohumeral joint stability. Clin Orthop Relat Res 1993;(291):20–8.

7. Halder AM, Kuhl SG, Zobitz ME, et al. Effects of the glenoid labrum and glenohumeral abduction on stability of the shoulder joint through concavity-compression: an in vitro study. J Bone Joint Surg Am 2001;83A(7):1062–9.

8. Matsen FA 3rd, Harryman DT 2nd, Sidles JA. Mechanics of glenohumeral instability. Clin Sports Med 1991;10(4):783–8.

9. Bankart AS. Recurrent or habitual dislocation of the shoulder-joint. Br Med J 1923; 2(3285):1132–3.

10. Taylor DC, Arciero RA. Pathologic changes associated with shoulder dislocations. Arthroscopic and physical examination findings in first-time, traumatic anterior dislocations. Am J Sports Med 1997;25(3):306–11.

11. Lazarus MD, Sidles JA, Harryman DT 2nd, et al. Effect of a chondral-labral defect on glenoid concavity and glenohumeral stability. A cadaveric model. J Bone Joint Surg Am 1996;78(1):94–102.

12. Owens BD, Nelson BJ, Duffey ML, et al. Pathoanatomy of first-time, traumatic, anterior glenohumeral subluxation events. J Bone Joint Surg Am 2010;92(7): 1605–11.

13. Lo IK, Parten PM, Burkhart SS. The inverted pear glenoid: an indicator of significant glenoid bone loss. Arthroscopy 2004;20(2):169–74.

14. Bigliani LU, Newton PM, Steinmann SP, et al. Glenoid rim lesions associated with recurrent anterior dislocation of the shoulder. Am J Sports Med 1998;26(1):41–5.

15. Itoi E, Lee SB, Berglund LJ, et al. The effect of a glenoid defect on anteroinferior stability of the shoulder after Bankart repair: a cadaveric study. J Bone Joint Surg Am 2000;82(1):35–46.

16. Burkhart SS, De Beer JF. Traumatic glenohumeral bone defects and their relationship to failure of arthroscopic Bankart repairs: significance of the inverted-pear glenoid and the humeral engaging Hill-Sachs lesion. Arthroscopy 2000;16(7): 677–94.

17. Piasecki DP, Verma NN, Romeo AA, et al. Glenoid bone deficiency in recurrent anterior shoulder instability: diagnosis and management. J Am Acad Orthop Surg 2009;17(8):482–93.

18. Headey J, Brooks JH, Kemp SP. The epidemiology of shoulder injuries in English professional rugby union. Am J Sports Med 2007;35(9):1537–43.

19. Owens BD, Duffey ML, Nelson BJ, et al. The incidence and characteristics of shoulder instability at the United States Military Academy. Am J Sports Med 2007;35(7):1168–73.

20. Ward JP, Bradley JP. Decision making in the in-season athlete with shoulder instability. Clin Sports Med 2013;32(4):685–96.

21. Arciero RA, Wheeler JH, Ryan JB, et al. Arthroscopic Bankart repair versus nonoperative treatment for acute, initial anterior shoulder dislocations. Am J Sports Med 1994;22(5):589–94.

22. Robinson CM, Howes J, Murdoch H, et al. Functional outcome and risk of recurrent instability after primary traumatic anterior shoulder dislocation in young patients. J Bone Joint Surg Am 2006;88(11):2326–36.

23. Sachs RA, Lin D, Stone ML, et al. Can the need for future surgery for acute traumatic anterior shoulder dislocation be predicted? J Bone Joint Surg Am 2007; 89(8):1665–74.

24. Robinson CM, Shur N, Sharpe T, et al. Injuries associated with traumatic anterior glenohumeral dislocations. J Bone Joint Surg Am 2012;94(1):18–26.

25. Safran O, Milgrom C, Radeva-Petrova DR, et al. Accuracy of the anterior apprehension test as a predictor of risk for redislocation after a first traumatic shoulder dislocation. Am J Sports Med 2010;38(5):972–5.

26. Lo IK, Nonweiler B, Woolfrey M, et al. An evaluation of the apprehension, relocation, and surprise tests for anterior shoulder instability. Am J Sports Med 2004; 32(2):301–7.

27. Jobe FW, Kvitne RS, Giangarra CE. Shoulder pain in the overhand or throwing athlete. The relationship of anterior instability and rotator cuff impingement. Orthop Rev 1989;18(9):963–75.

28. Hegedus EJ, Goode AP, Cook CE, et al. Which physical examination tests provide clinicians with the most value when examining the shoulder? Update of a systematic review with meta-analysis of individual tests. Br J Sports Med 2012; 46(14):964–78.

29. Tzannes A, Murrell GA. Clinical examination of the unstable shoulder. Sports Med 2002;32(7):447–57.

30. van Kampen DA, van den Berg T, van der Woude HJ, et al. Diagnostic value of patient characteristics, history, and six clinical tests for traumatic anterior shoulder instability. J Shoulder Elbow Surg 2013;22(10):1310–9.

31. Boileau P, Villalba M, Héry JY, et al. Risk factors for recurrence of shoulder instability after arthroscopic Bankart repair. J Bone Joint Surg Am 2006;88(8): 1755–63.

32. Balg F, Boileau P. The instability severity index score. A simple pre-operative score to select patients for arthroscopic or open shoulder stabilisation. J Bone Joint Surg Br 2007;89(11):1470–7.

33. Pavlov H, Warren RF, Weiss CB Jr, et al. The roentgenographic evaluation of anterior shoulder instability. Clin Orthop Relat Res 1985;(194):153–8.

34. Bois AJ, Walker RE, Kodali P, et al. Imaging instability in the athlete: the right modality for the right diagnosis. Clin Sports Med 2013;32(4):653–84.

35. Omoumi P, Teixeira P, Lecouvet F, et al. Glenohumeral joint instability. J Magn Reson Imaging 2011;33(1):2–16.

36. Hill HA, Sachs MD. The grooved defect of the humeral head. Radiology 1940; 35(6):690–700.

37. Yamamoto N, Itoi E, Abe H, et al. Contact between the glenoid and the humeral head in abduction, external rotation, and horizontal extension: a new concept of glenoid track. J Shoulder Elbow Surg 2007;16(5):649–56.

38. Owens BD, Burns TC, Campbell SE, et al. Simple method of glenoid bone loss calculation using ipsilateral magnetic resonance imaging. Am J Sports Med 2013;41(3):622–4.

39. Bhatia S, Saigal A, Frank RM, et al. Glenoid diameter is an inaccurate method for percent glenoid bone loss quantification: analysis and techniques for improved accuracy. Arthroscopy 2015;31(4):608–14.e1.

40. Itoi E, Hatakeyama Y, Kido T, et al. A new method of immobilization after traumatic anterior dislocation of the shoulder: a preliminary study. J Shoulder Elbow Surg 2003;12(5):413–5.

41. Hovelius L, Eriksson K, Fredin H, et al. Recurrences after initial dislocation of the shoulder. Results of a prospective study of treatment. J Bone Joint Surg Am 1983; 65(3):343–9.

42. Buss DD, Lynch GP, Meyer CP, et al. Nonoperative management for in-season athletes with anterior shoulder instability. Am J Sports Med 2004;32(6):1430–3.

43. Itoi E, Hatakeyama Y, Sato T, et al. Immobilization in external rotation after shoulder dislocation reduces the risk of recurrence. A randomized controlled trial. J Bone Joint Surg Am 2007;89(10):2124–31.

44. Itoi E, Sashi R, Minagawa H, et al. Position of immobilization after dislocation of the glenohumeral joint. A study with use of magnetic resonance imaging. J Bone Joint Surg Am 2001;83A(5):661–7.

45. Paterson WH, Throckmorton TW, Koester M, et al. Position and duration of immobilization after primary anterior shoulder dislocation: a systematic review and meta-analysis of the literature. J Bone Joint Surg Am 2010;92(18):2924–33.

46. Kuhn JE. Treating the initial anterior shoulder dislocation–an evidence-based medicine approach. Sports Med Arthrosc 2006;14(4):192–8.

47. Harris JD, Romeo AA. Arthroscopic management of the contact athlete with instability. Clin Sports Med 2013;32(4):709–30.

48. Wheeler JH, Ryan JB, Arciero RA, et al. Arthroscopic versus nonoperative treatment of acute shoulder dislocations in young athletes. Arthroscopy 1989;5(3): 213–7.

49. Mazzocca AD, Brown FM Jr, Carreira DS, et al. Arthroscopic anterior shoulder stabilization of collision and contact athletes. Am J Sports Med 2005;33(1):52–60.

50. Gerometta A, Rosso C, Klouche S, et al. Arthroscopic Bankart shoulder stabilization in athletes: return to sports and functional outcomes. Knee Surg Sports Traumatol Arthrosc 2016;24(6):1877–83.

51. Rice SG. Medical conditions affecting sports participation. American Academy of Pediatrics Committee on Sports Medicine and Fitness. Pediatrics 1994;94(5): 757–60.

52. Cho NS, Hwang JC, Rhee YG. Arthroscopic stabilization in anterior shoulder instability: collision athletes versus noncollision athletes. Arthroscopy 2006; 22(9):947–53.

53. Larrain MV, Montenegro HJ, Mauas DM, et al. Arthroscopic management of traumatic anterior shoulder instability in collision athletes: analysis of 204 cases with a 4- to 9-year follow-up and results with the suture anchor technique. Arthroscopy 2006;22(12):1283–9.

54. Levy O, Matthews T, Even T. The "purse-string" technique: an arthroscopic technique for stabilization of anteroinferior instability of the shoulder with early and medium-term results. Arthroscopy 2007;23(1):57–64.

55. Ozturk BY, Maak TG, Fabricant P, et al. Return to sports after arthroscopic anterior stabilization in patients aged younger than 25 years. Arthroscopy 2013;29(12): 1922–31.

56. Pagnani MJ, Warren RF, Altchek DW, et al. Arthroscopic shoulder stabilization using transglenoid sutures. A four-year minimum follow-up. Am J Sports Med 1996; 24(4):459–67.

57. Petrera M, Dwyer T, Tsuji MR, et al. Outcomes of arthroscopic Bankart repair in collision versus noncollision athletes. Orthopedics 2013;36(5):e621–6.

58. Roberts SN, Taylor DE, Brown JN, et al. Open and arthroscopic techniques for the treatment of traumatic anterior shoulder instability in Australian rules football players. J Shoulder Elbow Surg 1999;8(5):403–9.

59. Rhee YG, Ha JH, Cho NS. Anterior shoulder stabilization in collision athletes: arthroscopic versus open Bankart repair. Am J Sports Med 2006;34(6):979–85.

60. Cole BJ, L'Insalata J, Irrgang J, et al. Comparison of arthroscopic and open anterior shoulder stabilization. A two to six-year follow-up study. J Bone Joint Surg Am 2000;82A(8):1108–14.

61. Jobe FW, Giangarra CE, Kvitne RS, et al. Anterior capsulolabral reconstruction of the shoulder in athletes in overhand sports. Am J Sports Med 1991;19(5):428–34.

62. Uhorchak JM, Arciero RA, Huggard D, et al. Recurrent shoulder instability after open reconstruction in athletes involved in collision and contact sports. Am J Sports Med 2000;28(6):794–9.

63. Bigliani LU, Kurzweil PR, Schwartzbach CC, et al. Inferior capsular shift procedure for anterior-inferior shoulder instability in athletes. Am J Sports Med 1994; 22(5):578–84.

64. Pagnani MJ, Dome DC. Surgical treatment of traumatic anterior shoulder instability in american football players. J Bone Joint Surg Am 2002;84A(5):711–5.

65. Uchiyama Y, Hamada K, Miyazaki S, et al. Neer modified inferior capsular shift procedure for recurrent anterior instability of the shoulder in judokas. Am J Sports Med 2009;37(5):995–1002.

66. Fabre T, Abi-Chahla ML, Billaud A, et al. Long-term results with Bankart procedure: a 26-year follow-up study of 50 cases. J Shoulder Elbow Surg 2010; 19(2):318–23.

67. Stone GP, Pearsall AW. Return to play after open Bankart repair: a systematic review. Orthop J Sports Med 2014;2(2). 2325967114522960.

68. Neyton L, Young A, Dawidziak B, et al. Surgical treatment of anterior instability in rugby union players: clinical and radiographic results of the Latarjet-Patte procedure with minimum 5-year follow-up. J Shoulder Elbow Surg 2012;21(12):1721–7.

69. Hovelius L, Sandström B, Sundgren K, et al. One hundred eighteen Bristow-Latarjet repairs for recurrent anterior dislocation of the shoulder prospectively followed for fifteen years: study I–clinical results. J Shoulder Elbow Surg 2004;13(5): 509–16.
70. Dickens JF, Rue JH, Cameron KL, et al. Improved return to play in intercollegiate contact athletes following arthroscopic stabilization for anterior shoulder instability: a prospective multicenter study. Orlando (FL): American Orthopaedic Society for Sports Medicine; 2015.
71. Harris JD, Gupta AK, Mall NA, et al. Long-term outcomes after Bankart shoulder stabilization. Arthroscopy 2013;29(5):920–33.
72. An VV, Sivakumar BS, Phan K, et al. A systematic review and meta-analysis of clinical and patient-reported outcomes following two procedures for recurrent traumatic anterior instability of the shoulder: Latarjet procedure vs. Bankart repair. J Shoulder Elbow Surg 2016;25(5):853–63.

Return to Play After Shoulder Surgery in Throwers

Robert Thorsness, MD*, Jeremy A. Alland, MD,
Colin B. McCulloch, BA, Anthony Romeo, MD

KEYWORDS

- Baseball • Softball • Football • Javelin • Cricket

KEY POINTS

- Return to play after superior labral anterior to posterior (SLAP) repair is poor.
- Surgeons need to be cautious with SLAP repair indications in overhead athletes.
- Pitchers possess unique shoulder kinematics, and often possess physiologic adaptations that are not necessarily pathologic.
- Open biceps tenodesis is a reasonable alternative to SLAP repair in overhand athletes.

INTRODUCTION

The throwing athlete's shoulder is a unique, complex entity with challenges in both diagnosis and management. The shoulders in these athletes possess unique biomechanics and physiologic adaptations that are not necessarily pathologic. Due to the continued remodeling of the adolescent shoulder during development, these adaptations occur to both the soft tissue structures and bone, and are imperative to successful throwing mechanics. These physiologic adaptations make clinical management in these patients quite challenging, as a careful balance needs to be met with what is an optimal physiologic adaptation versus a pathologic condition that necessitates treatment. Because of this, return to play (RTP) outcomes are often poor when specifically evaluating overhead athletes. It is important to note that even though these athletes may demonstrate improvements in pain and general function following surgical management, subtle changes in accuracy or velocity as a result of surgery can significantly affect the success of an overhead throwing athlete at the competitive level.

Department of Orthopaedic Surgery, Rush University Medical Center, 1611 West Harrison Street, Suite 200, Chicago, IL 60612, USA
* Corresponding author. Department of Orthopaedic Surgery, Rush University Medical Center, 1611 West Harrison Street, Suite 200, Chicago, IL 60654.
E-mail address: Robert_j_thorsness@rush.edu

Clin Sports Med 35 (2016) 563–575
http://dx.doi.org/10.1016/j.csm.2016.05.003
0278-5919/16/$ – see front matter © 2016 Elsevier Inc. All rights reserved.

The biceps-labral complex (BLC) is a common source of pathology in overhead athletes and frequently includes pathology to the long head biceps tendon (LHBT) and superior labrum in the form of superior labral anterior to posterior (SLAP) tears, which are often managed with SLAP repair in overhead athletes, especially type II SLAP tears (**Fig. 1**).[1] Although SLAP tears can occur in isolation in these athletes, they more frequently coincide with other shoulder pathology, such as partial-thickness undersurface rotator cuff tears, biceps tendinitis, glenohumeral internal rotation deficit (GIRD), and anterior microinstability. Recently, there has been a noteworthy increase in the incidence and surgical treatment of SLAP tears.[2] Management of these patients needs to take into account the loads that will be placed on the shoulder postoperatively and the need for return to sport. Unfortunately, return to sport for overhead throwing athletes following SLAP repair is poor,[3,4] highlighting the need for appropriate surgical indications and possible alterations in surgical technique to improve RTP outcomes.

With regard to BLC lesions, the thrower's shoulder deserves special attention given its unique mechanics. Pitchers and other overhead athletes have high clinical expectations, often with goals of returning to high-level competition, emphasizing the need for proper diagnosis and management in these patients. The baseball pitch is the fastest described human motion, often exceeding 7000° per second. This places tremendous forces through the shoulder, and can exceed 1000 N in professional pitchers.[5] Some believe that the etiology of BLC lesions in these athletes involves tension during the deceleration phase of throwing, which can lead to both LHBT lesions as well as SLAP tears, or peel-back during the late-cocking phase of throwing. These lesions may be exacerbated by the presence of associated anterior microinstability or GIRD, and are often seen in combination with other shoulder pathology, such as rotator cuff tears.[6–8]

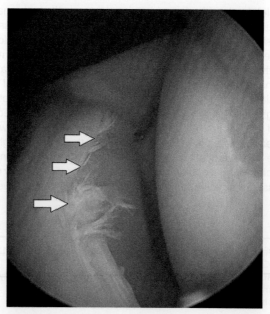

Fig. 1. LHBT and superior labral pathology is common in overhead athletes. View from posterior portal demonstrates a posterior-superior labral tear in an overhead athlete (*white arrows*).

Although RTP outcomes for SLAP repair are poor, biceps tenodesis as an alternative has demonstrated excellent clinical outcomes for patients with primary LHBT pathology as well as for failed SLAP repairs.[9–11] Although there are few data regarding clinical outcomes of primary biceps tenodesis in overhead athletes, we have been using this technique for patients who present with symptoms localized to the bicipital groove with good results.[12] The goals of the present article are to review the most common pathology that presents in overhead athletes and discuss the surgical management strategies to optimize their chances of RTP at their prior level of competition. Further, we review the optimal postoperative rehabilitation strategies for these athletes.

SUPERIOR LABRAL ANTERIOR TO POSTERIOR REPAIR

SLAP repair remains controversial in overhead athletes given that outcome studies are troubled by confounding variables and more importantly, these patients experience inconsistent RTP outcomes.[3,4] Further, some SLAP tears may actually be physiologic adaptations to throwing kinematics, as they are often asymptomatic in this population, further complicating decision making.[13] We advocate for SLAP repair in young overhead athletes with a consistent history, physical examination, and imaging, in the absence of LHBT symptoms or examination findings (**Fig. 2**).

When repairing an SLAP tear in a thrower's shoulder, the most common complication is inability to RTP. The etiology is likely multifactorial, including residual pain, loss of range of motion (ROM), failure of healing, hardware-related complications, and poor postoperative shoulder mechanics.[14]

In a retrospective cohort study, Neuman and colleagues[15] looked at the ability of throwers to return to their preinjury playing level after arthroscopic repair of a type II SLAP lesion. Of the 30 athletes included in this study, baseball/softball players returned to their preinjury level of play at lower rates (79.5%) compared with athletes of other overhead sports, including javelin and tennis (93.9%). In addition, the Kerlan-Jobe Orthopedic Clinic Shoulder and Elbow score (KJOC) was decreased in baseball/softball players compared with the other overhead sport athletes, even though the American Shoulder and Elbow Society (ASES) score was nearly identical (87.9 vs 87.8). This suggests that the KJOC score may provide a better prediction of a throwing

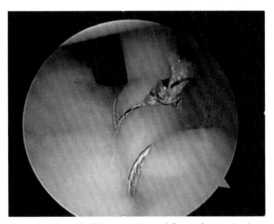

Fig. 2. SLAP repair in an overhand athlete as viewed from the posterior portal in the lateral decubitus position.

athlete's ability to RTP for throwers following arthroscopic repair of a type II SLAP lesion.

Cohen and colleagues[16] examined 23 professional baseball players' ability to RTP following a type II SLAP lesion treated surgically with no concomitant rotator cuff pathology. Twenty-two of the players underwent SLAP repair, and 1 player underwent debridement of a posterior labral flap tear. Of these players, 7 (31.8%) were able to return to the same level of play, 5 (22.7%) returned to a lower level, and 10 (45.4%) were unable to RTP and retired from professional baseball. The single player who underwent labral debridement returned to the same level of play.

Neri and colleagues[17] surveyed 23 elite athletes who had undergone surgical repair of a type II SLAP lesion at a mean follow-up of 38 months. The investigators found that only 57% of patients had returned to their preinjury level of competitiveness, 26% had returned to their sport but were limited by pain, and the remaining patients were unable to return to sport. A concomitant partial-thickness rotator cuff tear was found in 35% of the patients evaluated in this study. Interestingly, the presence of rotator cuff tear was predictive of a patient's ability to return to preinjury level of competition (12.5% in the group with rotator cuff tears vs 80% in the group without).

Park and colleagues[18] were the first to examine the use of bioabsorbable suture anchors in 24 elite overhead athletes being surgically treated for a type II SLAP lesion. Twelve of the patients (50%) were able to return to sport following surgery. In addition, a smaller percentage of patients who played baseball returned compared with all other overhand athletes in this study (38% vs 75%). Of the professional baseball players, only 2 of the 8 were able to reach their preinjury level of performance. In contrast, Ide and colleagues[19] evaluated the outcomes of 40 overhead athletes managed with SLAP repair and demonstrated better RTP outcomes. Among the athletes, 90% achieved a satisfactory result, with 75% returning to sport at the same level of competitiveness. Among the 19 baseball players, however, 12 (63%) were able to return to sport at the same level of competitiveness.

Kim and colleagues[20] evaluated the clinical outcomes in a population of 34 patients (16 nonoverhead sports and 18 overhead sports athletes) who underwent arthroscopic repair for a superior labral lesion. The investigators found that those who participated in overhead sports had significantly lower functional outcome scores compared with patients who did not participate in overhead sports. Among the overhead sport athletes and their return to preinjury sport participation and activities, 3 of the 18 patients had severe limitations, 3 of the patients had moderate limitations, and 8 had mild limitations. The remaining 4 patients had no limitations.

Recently, Fedoriw and colleagues[4] evaluated 45 professional pitchers and 23 professional position players who suffered from a type II SLAP tear for both RTP characteristics as well as their ability to return to prior level of performance (RPP). Among these players, those who failed 2 rehabilitation attempts or were unsatisfied after returning to play following rehabilitation (27 pitchers and 13 position players) were surgically treated. The overall RTP rate was 40%, and their RPP was 22%. Unfortunately, the RTP rate for the 27 pitchers following surgery was 48%, and the RPP rate was only 7%. The RTP rate for 13 position players following surgery was better at 85%, with an RPP rate of 54%. Of the 2 pitchers able to return to prior performance, both underwent labral debridement only instead of SLAP repair. These results highlight the often dismal RTP rates in high-performance overhead athletes, particularly pitchers, when managed with SLAP repair.

More encouraging RTP results were highlighted by Ricchetti and colleagues,[21] who were able to identify 51 pitchers who underwent isolated labral repair using the official team injury report from Major League Baseball (MLB) teams. Data from the 3 seasons before and after the labral repair were analyzed for the players and compared with a cohort of 110 randomly selected major league pitchers from the 2000 MLB season not known to have had labral or rotator cuff surgery. Of the 51 injured pitchers, 37 (72.5%) returned to play in a major league game at a mean of 13.1 months following surgery. Among the pitchers who returned to play following surgery there was no significant change in their mean innings pitched, earned run average, and walks and hits per inning pitched per year, suggesting no loss in performance. In addition, they noted that the greater the number of innings pitched per year preinjury was associated with an increased likelihood of returning to play in the major leagues.

Clearly, the results of RTP after SLAP repair are inconsistent, and often very poor in overhead athletes. A recent systematic review demonstrated an RTP rate of 64% after SLAP repair, with rates as low as 7% when evaluating overhead athletes.[3,4] Thus, the surgeon must remain realistic and discuss these potential outcomes with the athlete before proceeding with surgery. Although surgical technique strategies for SLAP repair are numerous, further research is necessary to determine the optimal technique for returning these athletes to competition.

LABRAL DEBRIDEMENT

Results following labral debridement as an alternative to SLAP repair in overhead athletes are lacking in the literature. Clearly, although the RTP outcomes for SLAP repair are often inconsistent, debridement can be successful in these athletes. Debridement alone, in theory, prevents the possible alteration in ROM and glenohumeral mechanics that could result as a consequence of SLAP repair in overhead athletes.

In a retrospective study, Martin and Garth[22] evaluated 24 patients with anterior or posterior glenoid labral tears managed with debridement alone. Patients with SLAP tears, however, were excluded. Long-term excellent clinical outcomes were observed in 21 patients (87.5%), with 16 patients (67%) returning to prior level of play. Among pitchers specifically, 62% were able to return to competition. In another retrospective study of 46 patients (30 baseball players) who underwent labral debridement for anteroinferior, anterosuperior, and posterior labral tears, Tomlinson and Glousman[23] demonstrated that 54% of patients had good to excellent results. Professional baseball players in particular had a significantly better outcome compared with nonprofessional players (75% good to excellent vs 43%, respectively). Good outcomes were defined as return to prior level of competition with mild pain, with excellent outcomes defined as return to prior level of competition with no pain.

Although labral debridement alone remains a viable option in particular players given the unpredictable RTP outcomes following SLAP repair, further study is needed to determine which players would benefit from this particular modality. Players with superior labral tears that are not amenable to repair could benefit from debridement versus biceps tenodesis.

OPEN BICEPS TENODESIS

No study to date has specifically evaluated the clinical outcomes or RTP characteristics of biceps tenodesis in overhead athletes, but several studies have included these patients within their cohorts. When indicated, we elect for open subpectoral biceps tenodesis with tenodesis screw fixation in overhead throwing athletes so as to achieve strong fixation of the tendon and to prevent the possibility of residual bicipital groove pain postoperatively. Tenotomy alone is not optimal in these athletes given concern for possible Popeye deformity and the potential for biceps muscle cramping postoperatively.

Primary tenodesis of the LHBT is an effective alternative treatment for SLAP tears in patients with concomitant biceps tendinitis.[9,12,24] Gupta and colleagues[12] evaluated 28 patients including 7 overhead athletes with symptomatic SLAP tears and biceps tendinitis that underwent primary open subpectoral biceps tenodesis. There was a significant improvement in outcome scores, and patients expressed good satisfaction postoperatively. Among the overhead athletes, RTP data were available for 5 of the 7 patients. Among these 5 patients, 3 (60%) returned to full previous level of play, 1 (20%) returned to a lower level of play, and 1 (20%) was unable to return due to continued pain.

In a nonrandomized prospective study conducted by Boileau and colleagues,[9] 2 groups of patients with isolated type II SLAP lesions underwent surgery: 10 patients (7 overhead athletes) underwent SLAP repair and 15 patients (8 overhead athletes) underwent arthroscopic biceps tenodesis with an interface screw. The mean age for patients in the SLAP repair and biceps tenodesis groups was 37 and 52 years, respectively, which was a significant difference. Of the 10 patients who underwent SLAP repair, 6 (60%) were dissatisfied with their results. In contrast, only 1 (7%) of the 15 patients in the biceps tenodesis group was dissatisfied. Notably, the biceps tenodesis group demonstrated a significantly better return to sport rate compared with the SLAP repair group (87% vs 20%, respectively). These results need to be interpreted with caution, as the group assignments were not randomized, and the decision for SLAP repair was based solely on patient age.

In contrast to the previously discussed study, Ek and colleagues[24] retrospectively compared patients undergoing SLAP repair and biceps tenodesis for type II SLAP tears and found no significant difference between the 2 treatment groups with regard to clinical outcome scores or return to sport. These cohorts also demonstrated a significant difference in age. This study, however, did not specifically comment on outcomes in overhead athletes.

Although the previously discussed clinical outcomes regarding SLAP repair and biceps tenodesis in these athletes may be equivocal, there is some biomechanical data suggesting that tenodesis may be superior. A recent motion analysis study by Chalmers and colleagues[14] has demonstrated that pitchers who undergo open biceps tenodesis (OBT) have more physiologic pitching mechanics when compared with pitchers who undergo SLAP repair. In this study, the investigators evaluated the differences between neuromuscular control and upper extremity motion during the overhead pitch in 3 groups of pitchers: an uninjured control group of pitchers, those who had had an SLAP repair, and those who had undergone a subpectoral biceps tenodesis. They demonstrated that compared with the uninjured group, both the SLAP repair group and tenodesis group demonstrated lower ball velocity, but the difference in velocity between the SLAP repair group and tenodesis group was not significant. Based on the surface electromyographic measurements that were taken during the pitching motion, there were no major kinematic differences among the different groups except for significantly altered patterns of thoracic rotation in the pitchers who had undergone an SLAP repair. It was also noted that tenodesis was better than SLAP repair at restoring the natural muscular activation pattern within the long head of the biceps.

Biceps tenodesis also does not appear to have any significant adverse effects on glenohumeral stability in the presence of an SLAP tear.[25] Clearly, although OBT may be an appropriate treatment for patients with SLAP tears and coexisting biceps tendinitis,[12] and early studies suggest that biceps tenodesis may be optimal for returning the overhead athlete to competition and restore more physiologic pitching mechanics, further study is needed to determine the appropriate surgical management strategy in overhead athletes.

GLENOHUMERAL INTERNAL ROTATION DEFICIT AND ANTERIOR MICROINSTABILITY

The overhead athlete's shoulder experiences many cycles of microtraumatic stresses that can attenuate the anterior soft tissues, making subtle anterior instability common in these athletes. However, it is imperative to remember that anterior laxity may be a physiologic adaptation in these athletes, and that aggressive capsulorrhaphy will likely impair an athlete's ability to throw given the limitations in ROM postoperatively. Although most overhead athletes will not present with frank instability, anterior microinstability can present with isolated pain in these patients.[26] Careful attention should be paid to GIRD in the overhead athlete, which is associated with anterior microinstability, posterior capsular tightness, partial undersurface rotator cuff tears, and SLAP lesions.[27–31]

Jones and colleagues[32] found encouraging results in the overhead athlete's ability to RTP following arthroscopic capsular plication for microtraumatic anterior instability related to isolated capsular redundancy. Of the 20 patients included in this study, 12 were treated with suture plication and 8 underwent suture anchor fixation. During examination under anesthesia, all patients were found to have significant anterior shoulder instability in addition to a redundant anterior capsule and a positive drive-through sign. Eighteen patients (90%) were able to return to overhead sports, with 17 patients returning to their preinjury level of play, at a mean follow-up of 3.6 years. No statistically significant difference was found in the RTP rate between the suture plication and suture anchor fixation groups. One patient from each group was unable to RTP, both of which had concomitant partial-thickness rotator cuff tears.

In an evaluation of 25 overhand throwing athletes, Jobe and colleagues[27] demonstrated that an anterior capsulolabral reconstruction can have good results in the presence of anterior microinstability. At a mean follow-up of 39 months, all but 1 athlete completed a formal rehabilitation program and results were rated excellent in 68%, good in 24%, fair in 4%, and poor in 4%. Seventeen (68%) patients returned to their prior competitive level for at least 1 year.

Regarding GIRD, the standard of care is nonoperative with a focus on posterior capsular stretching. A posterior-inferior capsular stretching program has been shown to return approximately 90% of athletes to play.[33] When this fails, a controversial surgical management strategy is posterior capsular release in overhead athletes. Yoneda and colleagues[34] evaluated 16 overhead throwing athletes after arthroscopic posterior-inferior capsular release. Among the cohort, 11 patients (69%) returned to their preinjury level of play, whereas the remaining 5 patients returned to a lower level of play. There was no evidence of iatrogenic instability postoperatively. In a similar study, Codding and colleagues[35] evaluated 13 overhead throwing athletes who underwent arthroscopic posterior-inferior capsular release for GIRD. Ten (77%) of 13 patients returned to their preoperative level of play or higher. ASES scores were significantly improved, and internal rotation was significantly increased in these patients.

Although these studies suggest that posterior-inferior capsular release may play a role in select patients, we cannot advocate for this procedure in light of the high success rate of nonoperative treatment, and the lack of high-level studies validating outcomes.

ROTATOR CUFF TEARS IN THE THROWING ATHLETE

Surgical management of rotator cuff tears in throwers is not ideal with regard to RTP, as clinical outcomes of both debridement and repair show that many throwers do not return to previous levels of competition. Among athletes who do undergo surgery, the outcomes are highly dependent on the extent of the rotator cuff lesion. A partial-thickness tear requiring debridement has far better outcomes than a full-thickness tear requiring repair.

Payne and colleagues[36] evaluated 43 athletes younger than 40 years with partial-thickness rotator cuff tears treated with debridement alone and subacromial decompression. The study included 29 overhead throwers with insidious-onset, atraumatic rotator cuff tears. At 2 years of follow-up, only 45% of the overhead throwers returned to preinjury sports. Fortunately, the results of Reynolds and colleagues[37] were more encouraging. They reviewed 82 professional pitchers with small partial-thickness rotator cuff tears treated with debridement alone. Of the 67 athletes with adequate follow-up data, 76% returned to some level of professional pitching, and 55% returned to the same or higher level of competition.

Ide and colleagues[38] were the first to include overhead throwers in their results of a transtendon repair for partial-thickness articular-sided rotator cuff tears. They evaluated 6 athletes, and at a mean follow-up of 39 months, 2 (33%) of the 6 returned to the same level of play or higher, whereas 3 (50%) returned to a lower level of play. Similarly, Conway[39] demonstrated success with repair of partial-thickness rotator cuff tears in 14 overhead throwing athletes. All of the athletes in this cohort had associated SLAP tears and 50% had anterior instability. Eight (89%) of the 9 patients were able to RTP at the same level or higher, whereas the last player returned to throwing but was unable to achieve preoperative velocity.

Unfortunately, full-thickness rotator cuff tears in overhead throwing athletes have a poor prognosis following repair. Tibone and colleagues[40] evaluated the outcomes of open acromioplasty and repair of partial and complete rotator cuff tears in 29 overhead throwing athletes, of whom only 41% were able to RTP at the same level. Within this population, there were 5 professional pitchers with full-thickness rotator cuff tears that were repaired. Only 2 of these athletes were able to return to professional pitching. More recently, Mazoue and Andrews[41] evaluated 12 professional pitchers and 2 professional positional players with full-thickness rotator cuff tears who underwent mini-open rotator cuff repair. At a mean follow-up of 66 months, only 1 pitcher and 1 position player were able to return to professional baseball.

RETURN TO SPORT IN ELITE PITCHERS

In a recent systematic review, Harris and colleagues[42] evaluated the return to sport following shoulder surgery in elite pitchers, including 287 athletes of whom most were MLB players. Surgical management included SLAP repair or debridement (46%), rotator cuff repair or debridement (35%), and thermal capsulorrhaphy (11%) with or without subacromial decompression. The overall rate of return to sport for the athletes was 68%, with a mean time to return to sport of 12 months. Performance tended to decrease before surgery for the athletes, but performance gradually improved postoperatively, although not reaching preinjury levels of pitching. One study reported on maximum velocity before and after surgery (debridement of partial-thickness rotator cuff tears), and demonstrated a mean decrease in velocity from 94.2 mph to 90.1 mph.[37] Unfortunately, due to concurrent diagnoses, the investigators were unable to compare return to sport for the varying surgical techniques and diagnoses, but the study does offer considerable insight into expectations when treating elite pitchers.[42]

RETURN TO THROWING

It is imperative that the throwing athlete follow a specific return-to-throwing rehabilitation program to decrease the risk of reinjury. Most reinjuries occur due to fatigue and

Table 1
Return-to-throwing protocol

45′ Phase	60′ Phase	90′ Phase	120′ Phase	150′ Phase	180′ Phase
Step 1	**Step 3**	**Step 5**	**Step 7**	**Step 9**	**Step 11**
A. Warm-up throwing	A. Warm-up throwing	A. Warm-up throwing	A. Warm-up throwing	A. Warm-up throwing	A. Warm-up throwing
B. 45′ throws (25 total)	B. 60′ throws (25 total)	B. 90′ throws (25 total)	B. 120′ throws (25 total)	B. 150′ throws (25 total)	B. 180′ throws (25 total)
C. Rest 5–10 min	C. Rest 5–10 min	C. Rest 5–10 min	C. Rest 5–10 min	C. Rest 5–10 min	C. Rest 5–10 min
D. Warm-up throwing	D. Warm-up throwing	D. Warm-up throwing	D. Warm-up throwing	D. Warm-up throwing	D. Warm-up throwing
E. 45′ throws (25 total)	E. 60′ throws (25 total)	E. 90′ throws (25 total)	E. 120′ throws (25 total)	E. 150′ throws (25 total)	E. 180′ throws (25 total)
Step 2	**Step 4**	**Step 6**	**Step 8**	**Step 10**	**Step 12**
A. Warm-up throwing	A. Warm-up throwing	A. Warm-up throwing	A. Warm-up throwing	A. Warm-up throwing	A. Warm-up throwing
B. 45′ throws (25 total)	B. 60′ throws (25 total)	B. 90′ throws (25 total)	B. 120′ throws (25 total)	B. 150′ throws (25 total)	B. 180′ throws (25 total)
C. Rest 5–10 min	C. Rest 5–10 min	C. Rest 5–10 min	C. Rest 5–10 min	C. Rest 5–10 min	C. Rest 5–10 min
D. Warm-up throwing	D. Warm-up throwing	D. Warm-up throwing	D. Warm-up throwing	D. Warm-up throwing	D. Warm-up throwing
E. 45′ throws (25 total)	E. 60′ throws (25 total)	E. 90′ throws (25 total)	E. 120′ throws (25 total)	E. 150′ throws (25 total)	E. 180′ throws (25 total)
F. Rest 5–10 min	F. Rest 5–10 min	F. Rest 5–10 min	F. Rest 5–10 min	F. Rest 5–10 min	F. Rest 5–10 min
G. Warm-up throwing	G. Warm-up throwing	G. Warm-up throwing	G. Warm-up throwing	G. Warm-up throwing	G. Warm-up throwing
H. 45′ throws (25 total)	H. 60′ throws (25 total)	H. 90′ throws (25 total)	H. 120′ throws (25 total)	H. 150′ throws (25 total)	H. 180′ throws (25 total)
					Step 13
					A. Return to position or pitching-specific program

Perform each step 2 to 3 times with minimum 1-day rest between sessions.
Progression to the next step occurs with pain-free throwing and stable mechanics.

an associated change in throwing mechanics. Most athletes are competitive by nature and may attempt to accelerate the intensity of the program too quickly. This increases the risk of reinjury and highlights the importance of adopting an interval throwing program.

The interval throwing program we recommend (**Table 1**) allows for individual variability, as each athlete will progress at a different rate. Each step begins with a warm-up at approximately 30 to 45 feet with progression to the target distance. The program is designed to throw at each step 2 to 3 times without pain or symptoms before progressing to the next step. It is important to supervise the athlete at each step to stress proper mechanics. At the end of the program, positional players should return to game situations at 50% and gradually increase to 100%. Pitchers should begin the return-to-pitching program (**Table 2**)

Throughout the program, the thrower must maintain pain-free motion and proper mechanics. The soreness rules (**Box 1**) can be used to evaluate the thrower after each step. If the thrower ever experiences pain, throwing should be stopped immediately. This is followed by a period of rest until pain-free throwing returns. Recurrent pain should be reevaluated by a physician. In addition to a throwing program, the thrower must continue with a maintenance exercise program. Specific exercises will vary based on the individual. At minimum, this includes rotator cuff strengthening, scapular stabilization, and posterior capsular stretching.

Table 2
Return-to-pitching protocol

Stage 1: Fastballs Only: All Pitches Are from Mound	Stage 2: Fastballs Only: All Pitches Are from Mound	Stage 3: Add Breaking Balls: All Pitches Are from Mound
Step 1	Step 9	Step 12
A. Interval program to 120′	A. Warm-up	A. Warm-up
B. 15 pitches at 50%	B. 60 pitches at 75%	B. 30 pitches at 75%
Step 2	C. 15 pitches in batting	C. 15 pitches at 50% -
A. Interval program to 120′	practice	breaking balls
B. 30 pitches at 50%	Step 10	Step 13
Step 3	A. Warm-up	A. Warm-up
A. Interval program to 120′	B. 50–60 pitches at 75%	B. 30 pitches at 75%
B. 45 pitches at 50%	C. 30 pitches in batting	C. 30 pitches at 75% -
Step 4	practice	breaking balls
A. Interval program to 120′	Step 11	D. 30 pitches in batting
B. 60 pitches at 50%	A. Warm-up	practice
Step 5	B. 45–50 pitches at 75%	Step 14
A. Interval program to 120′	C. 45 pitches in batting	A. Warm-up
B. 70 pitches at 50%	practice	B. 30 pitches at 75%
Step 6		C. 60–90 pitches in batting
A. Interval program to 120′		practice, gradually
B. 45 pitches at 50%		increase breaking balls
C. 30 pitches at 75%		Step 15
Step 7		A. Simulated game
A. Interval program to 120′		B. Progress by 15 pitches each
B. 30 pitches at 50%		session
C. 45 pitches at 75%		
Step 8		
A. Interval program to 120′		
B. 65 pitches at 75%		
C. 10 pitches at 50%		

Perform each step 1 to 2 times with 1 day rest between sessions.
Progression to next step is based on the soreness rules.

Box 1
Soreness rules

A. If no soreness, advance steps per throwing program

B. If sore during warm-up but soreness is gone within the first 15 throws, repeat the previous workout. If shoulder becomes sore during this workout, stop and take 2 days off. On return to throwing, drop down 1 step.

C. If sore more than 1 hour after throwing, or the next day, take 1 day off and repeat the most recent throwing program workout.

D. If sore during warm-up and soreness continues through the first 15 throws, stop throwing and take 2 days off. On return to throwing, drop down 1 step.

SUMMARY

The throwing athlete's shoulder is a unique, complex entity with challenges in both diagnosis and management. The shoulders in these athletes possess unique biomechanics and pathologic conditions. Unfortunately, RTP outcomes are often poor when specifically evaluating overhead athletes, especially with regard to SLAP repair. There may be a role for OBT in these athletes, but further research is needed to validate the outcomes of this procedure. It is imperative for the surgeon to be cautious when indicating these athletes for surgery, because although they may demonstrate improvements in pain and general function, subtle changes in accuracy or velocity as a result of surgery can significantly affect the success of an overhead throwing athlete at the competitive level.

REFERENCES

1. Snyder SJ, Karzel RP, Del Pizzo W, et al. SLAP lesions of the shoulder. Arthroscopy 1990;6:274–9.

2. Weber SC, Martin DF, Seiler JG, et al. Superior labrum anterior and posterior lesions of the shoulder: incidence rates, complications, and outcomes as reported by American Board of Orthopedic Surgery. Part II candidates. Am J Sports Med 2012;40:1538–43.

3. Gorantla K, Gill C, Wright RW. The outcome of type II SLAP repair: a systematic review. Arthroscopy 2010;26:537–45.

4. Fedoriw WW, Ramkumar P, McCulloch PC, et al. Return to play after treatment of superior labral tears in professional baseball players. Am J Sports Med 2014;42: 1155–60.

5. Fleisig GS, Andrews JR, Dillman CJ, et al. Kinetics of baseball pitching with implications about injury mechanisms. Am J Sports Med 1995;23:233–9.

6. Andrews JR, Carson WG Jr, McLeod WD. Glenoid labrum tears related to the long head of the biceps. Am J Sports Med 1985;13:337–41.

7. Bey MJ, Elders GJ, Huston LJ, et al. The mechanism of creation of superior labrum, anterior, and posterior lesions in a dynamic biomechanical model of the shoulder: the role of inferior subluxation. J Shoulder Elbow Surg 1998;7: 397–401.

8. Burkhart SS, Morgan CD, Kibler WB. Shoulder injuries in overhead athletes. The "dead arm" revisited. Clin Sports Med 2000;19:125–58.

9. Boileau P, Parratte S, Chuinard C, et al. Arthroscopic treatment of isolated type II SLAP lesions: biceps tenodesis as an alternative to reinsertion. Am J Sports Med 2009;37:929–36.

10. Gupta AK, Bruce B, Klosterman EL, et al. Subpectoral biceps tenodesis for failed type II SLAP repair. Orthopedics 2013;36:e723–8.

11. Mazzocca AD, Cote MP, Arciero CL, et al. Clinical outcomes after subpectoral biceps tenodesis with an interference screw. Am J Sports Med 2008;36:1922–9.

12. Gupta AK, Chalmers PN, Klosterman EL, et al. Subpectoral biceps tenodesis for bicipital tendonitis with SLAP tear. Orthopedics 2015;38:e48–53.

13. Lesniak BP, Baraga MG, Jose J, et al. Glenohumeral findings on magnetic resonance imaging correlate with innings pitched in asymptomatic pitchers. Am J Sports Med 2013;41:2022–7.

14. Chalmers PN, Trombley R, Cip J, et al. Postoperative restoration of upper extremity motion and neuromuscular control during the overhand pitch: evaluation of tenodesis and repair for superior labral anterior-posterior tears. Am J Sports Med 2014;42:2825–36.

15. Neuman BJ, Boisvert CB, Reiter B, et al. Results of arthroscopic repair of type II superior labral anterior posterior lesions in overhead athletes: assessment of return to preinjury playing level and satisfaction. Am J Sports Med 2011;39:1883–8.

16. Cohen SB, Sheridan S, Ciccotti MG. Return to sports for professional baseball players after surgery of the shoulder or elbow. Sports Health 2011;3:105–11.

17. Neri BR, ElAttrache NS, Owsley KC, et al. Outcome of type II superior labral anterior posterior repairs in elite overhead athletes: Effect of concomitant partial-thickness rotator cuff tears. Am J Sports Med 2011;39:114–20.

18. Park JY, Chung SW, Jeon SH, et al. Clinical and radiological outcomes of type 2 superior labral anterior posterior repairs in elite overhead athletes. Am J Sports Med 2013;41:1372–9.

19. Ide J, Maeda S, Takagi K. Sports activity after arthroscopic superior labral repair using suture anchors in overhead-throwing athletes. Am J Sports Med 2005;33: 507–14.

20. Kim SH, Ha KI, Kim SH, et al. Results of arthroscopic treatment of superior labral lesions. J Bone Joint Surg Am 2002;84-A:981–5.

21. Ricchetti ET, Weidner Z, Lawrence JT, et al. Glenoid labral repair in Major League Baseball pitchers. Int J Sports Med 2010;31:265–70.

22. Martin DR, Garth WP Jr. Results of arthroscopic debridement of glenoid labral tears. Am J Sports Med 1995;23:447–51.

23. Tomlinson RJ Jr, Glousman RE. Arthroscopic debridement of glenoid labral tears in athletes. Arthroscopy 1995;11:42–51.

24. Ek ET, Shi LL, Tompson JD, et al. Surgical treatment of isolated type II superior labrum anterior-posterior (SLAP) lesions: repair versus biceps tenodesis. J Shoulder Elbow Surg 2014;23:1059–65.

25. Strauss EJ, Salata MJ, Sershon RA, et al. Role of the superior labrum after biceps tenodesis in glenohumeral stability. J Shoulder Elbow Surg 2014;23:485–91.

26. Glousman RE. Instability versus impingement syndrome in the throwing athlete. Orthop Clin North Am 1993;24:89–99.

27. Jobe FW, Giangarra CE, Kvitne RS, et al. Anterior capsulolabral reconstruction of the shoulder in athletes in overhand sports. Am J Sports Med 1991;19:428–34.

28. Jobe FW, Kvitne RS, Giangarra CE. Shoulder pain in the overhand or throwing athlete. The relationship of anterior instability and rotator cuff impingement. Orthop Rev 1989;18:963–75.

29. Kvitne RS, Jobe FW. The diagnosis and treatment of anterior instability in the throwing athlete. Clin Orthop Relat Res 1993;107–23.
30. Kvitne RS, Jobe FW, Jobe CM. Shoulder instability in the overhand or throwing athlete. Clin Sports Med 1995;14:917–35.
31. Reinold MM, Gill TJ, Wilk KE, et al. Current concepts in the evaluation and treatment of the shoulder in overhead throwing athletes, part 2: injury prevention and treatment. Sports Health 2010;2:101–15.
32. Jones KJ, Kahlenberg CA, Dodson CC, et al. Arthroscopic capsular plication for microtraumatic anterior shoulder instability in overhead athletes. Am J Sports Med 2012;40:2009–14.
33. Burkhart SS, Morgan CD, Kibler WB. The disabled throwing shoulder: spectrum of pathology Part I: pathoanatomy and biomechanics. Arthroscopy 2003;19:404–20.
34. Yoneda M, Nakagawa S, Mizuno N, et al. Arthroscopic capsular release for painful throwing shoulder with posterior capsular tightness. Arthroscopy 2006;22:801.e1–5.
35. Codding J, Dahm DL, McCarty LP 3rd, et al. Arthroscopic posterior-inferior capsular release in the treatment of overhead athletes. Am J Orthop (Belle Mead NJ) 2015;44:223–7.
36. Payne LZ, Altchek DW, Craig EV, et al. Arthroscopic treatment of partial rotator cuff tears in young athletes. A preliminary report. Am J Sports Med 1997;25:299–305.
37. Reynolds SB, Dugas JR, Cain EL, et al. Debridement of small partial-thickness rotator cuff tears in elite overhead throwers. Clin Orthop Relat Res 2008;466:614–21.
38. Ide J, Maeda S, Takagi K. Arthroscopic transtendon repair of partial-thickness articular-side tears of the rotator cuff: anatomical and clinical study. Am J Sports Med 2005;33:1672–9.
39. Conway JE. Arthroscopic repair of partial-thickness rotator cuff tears and SLAP lesions in professional baseball players. Orthop Clin North Am 2001;32:443–56.
40. Tibone JE, Elrod B, Jobe FW, et al. Surgical treatment of tears of the rotator cuff in athletes. J Bone Joint Surg Am 1986;68:887–91.
41. Mazoue CG, Andrews JR. Repair of full-thickness rotator cuff tears in professional baseball players. Am J Sports Med 2006;34:182–9.
42. Harris JD, Frank JM, Jordan MA, et al. Return to sport following shoulder surgery in the elite pitcher: a systematic review. Sports Health 2013;5:367–76.

Return to Play Following Ulnar Collateral Ligament Reconstruction

Edward Lyle Cain Jr, MD*, Owen McGonigle, MD

KEYWORDS

- UCL • UCL tear • UCL reconstruction • Outcomes after UCL reconstruction
- Return to play after UCL reconstruction • UCL rehab • UCL complications

KEY POINTS

- The incidence of Ulnar collateral ligament (UCL) surgery has been increasing particularly in younger athletes involved in year-round pitching for multiple teams without well-defined and enforced pitch counts.
- A standardized evaluation of athletes with medial elbow pain including thorough history, comprehensive physical examination and appropriate imaging studies are essential to make the diagnosis of UCL tear.
- There have been several surgical techniques described for UCL reconstruction, many of which have had good to excellent results in returning overhead throwing athletes back to their sport.
- Transient ulnar neuritis is the most common postoperative complication and is relatively common. Major complications are relatively rare and include need for revision UCL reconstruction and fracture.

INTRODUCTION

Nontraumatic ulnar collateral ligament (UCL) injury is most commonly seen in overhead athletes, with baseball pitchers at the highest risk of developing UCL insufficiency. UCL dysfunction typically presents as pain with loss of velocity and control. Some patients will present with an acute injury, whereas many will report a more insidious onset of symptoms with progressive pain with throwing and decreased performance. Treatment ranges from nonoperative rehabilitation to ligament reconstruction. Reports show overall good return to previous level of competition in those who undergo surgery.[1] Recently, investigators have documented a significant rise in these elbow injuries in young athletes, especially pitchers.[2]

Andrews Sports Medicine and Orthopaedic Center, American Sports Medicine Institute, 805 St. Vincent's Drive, Suite 100, Birmingham, AL 35205, USA
* Corresponding author.
E-mail address: lyle.cain@andrewscenters.com

Clin Sports Med 35 (2016) 577–595
http://dx.doi.org/10.1016/j.csm.2016.05.004
0278-5919/16/$ – see front matter © 2016 Elsevier Inc. All rights reserved.

ANATOMY AND BIOMECHANICS OF THE ULNAR COLLATERAL LIGAMENT

The UCL provides the primary restraint to valgus stress at the elbow. Its 3 main components are the oblique, posterior, and anterior bundles.[3] The oblique bundle, or transverse ligament, both originates and inserts on the ulna and does not provide true stability to the elbow joint.[4] The posterior bundle is a fan-shaped thickening of the capsule that provides minimal, if any, stability to the elbow.[4] The anterior bundle provides the main valgus restraint in the pitching motion and is the main restraint to valgus stress from 30 to 120° of elbow motion.[5] The anterior bundle originates on the anteroinferior edge of the medial humeral epicondyle (**Fig. 1**), with a mean footprint of 45.5 mm^2 and inserts an average of 2.8 mm distal to the ulna articular margin (**Fig. 2**), with a mean footprint length of 29.2 mm on the sublime tubercle of the ulna[5] (**Fig. 3**). The mean length of the UCL is 53.9 mm, with a mean width of 5.8 to 9.2 mm.[5] The anterior bundle inserts onto the sublime tubercle with a ridge that separates the bundle into anterior and posterior bands of equal size. The anterior band of the anterior bundle provides primary valgus restraint especially at 60° to 90° of flexion and its repair is crucial to adequate reconstruction.[4] The posterior band of the UCL provides secondary restraint to valgus force at the elbow at 90 to 120° of elbow flexion.[4]

Biomechanical studies have shown valgus forces at the elbow to be as high as 64 Newton-meters (N-m) during the late cocking and acceleration phases of throwing.[6] Varus torque moments are needed to counteract these forces and are typically generated from the UCL, flexor-pronator muscles, capsular tissue, and bony constraints of the elbow joint. Morrey and An[7] determined in a cadaver model that the UCL generated 54% of the resistance to a valgus force with the elbow at 90° of flexion. During active pitching, this value is likely reduced due to simultaneous muscle contraction, but if one assumes the UCL bears 54% of the maximal load, the UCL must be able to withstand 34 N-m. The UCL can withstand a maximum valgus torque between 22.7 and 34 N-m[6]; therefore, during pitching, the UCL frequently is at or above its failure load.

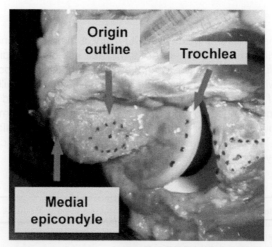

Fig. 1. The origin of the UCL has been carefully dissected from its bony attachment. Its outline has been marked. There is no attachment to the trochlea. (*From* Dugas JR, Ostrander RV, Cain EL, et al. Anatomy of the anterior bundle of the ulnar collateral ligament. J Shoulder Elbow Surg 2007;16(5):658; with permission.)

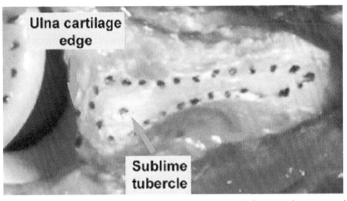

Fig. 2. The insertion of the UCL has been carefully dissected from its bony attachment. Its outline has been marked. Note the separation between the ulna cartilage edge and the proximal insertion. (*From* Dugas JR, Ostrander RV, Cain EL, et al. Anatomy of the anterior bundle of the ulnar collateral ligament. J Shoulder Elbow Surg 2007;16(5):659; with permission.)

RISK FACTORS FOR ULNAR COLLATERAL LIGAMENT INJURY

The incidence of UCL surgery has been shown to be increasing over time. Erickson and colleagues[2] found that patients in the 15-year-old to 19-year-old age group not only accounted for most patients undergoing surgery but that the number of procedures was also growing fastest in this group with an average increase of 9.12% per year. Much attention recently has been paid to the cause of the increasing number of UCL injuries, particularly in younger pitchers. Fleisig and Andrews[8] found that extended seasons, higher pitch counts, year-round pitching, pitching while fatigued, and pitching for multiple teams are risk factors for elbow injuries.[8] Pitchers who also play catcher are at a higher risk due to more total throws than those who pitch and play other positions or pitch only.[8] In a study of adolescent baseball pitchers, Olsen and colleagues[9] found a similar correlation between pitching volume and injury. They also noted that those who were injured tended to throw with higher velocity

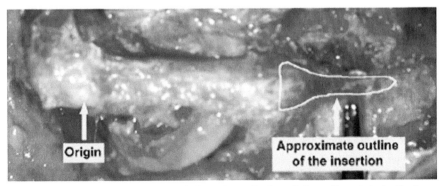

Fig. 3. The anterior bundle is exposed along its entire length from the origin to the insertion. The approximate insertion is outlined. (*From* Dugas JR, Ostrander RV, Cain EL, et al. Anatomy of the anterior bundle of the ulnar collateral ligament. J Shoulder Elbow Surg 2007;16(5):658; with permission.)

and were taller and heavier than a matched uninjured group. These same pitchers were more likely to pitch in showcases, pitch for multiple teams, and pitch with pain and fatigue than their uninjured peers[9] (**Box 1**). Pitchers in the southern United States, where baseball is more likely to be played year round, are also more likely to undergo UCL reconstruction than those from the northern states.[10]

PATIENT EVALUATION

A standard evaluation with a history, physical examination, and imaging is completed in all throwers with elbow pain. Cain and colleagues[1] found that 100% of patients experienced pain during athletic activity and that 96% of throwers complained of pain during late cocking and early acceleration phases of the throwing motion. Nearly half reported an acute onset of pain, and 53% were unable to identify a single inciting event. Seventy-five percent of the acute injuries were during competition. Delayed diagnosis was common, with an average time to diagnosis after onset of symptoms of 6.4 months. Neurologic symptoms were seen in 23% of athletes, most of which were ulnar nerve paresthesias during throwing.[1]

Physical examination of the athlete with concern for UCL injury should start with inspection. Unless the patient presents with an acute injury, there is often no significant swelling or outward signs of trauma. Range of motion may be somewhat decreased in this population. Cain and colleagues[1] found range of motion (ROM) at presentation in their series of UCL injuries averaged 5 to 135° with 85° of supination and pronation. Palpation over the origin of the UCL on the medial epicondyle and insertion on the sublime tubercle may reproduce pain. It is important to palpate all major bony and soft tissue structures as part of the examination as well to evaluate for concomitant injuries about the elbow. The UCL can be stressed by inducing a valgus stress at 30° of elbow flexion to unlock the bony congruity. This may reproduce symptoms of pain or laxity; however, even in compete UCL tears the amount of laxity may be too small to detect a side-to-side difference.[11] The milking maneuver is used to assess UCL stability at greater than 90° of flexion in the position of throwing. With the shoulder abducted to 90°, the elbow flexed to 90°, and the forearm supinated, the examiner pulls posteriorly on the examiner's thumb[11] (**Fig. 4**). A positive test elicits pain most frequently but instability and apprehension also may be elicited. The moving valgus stress test is performed in a similar position but the elbow begins in a fully flexed position and is brought from flexion to extension with a positive test provoking the most significant pain between 120° and 70° of flexion.[12] A valgus extension overload test[11] should

---

Box 1
Recommendations for adolescent baseball pitchers

1. Avoid pitching with arm pain

2. Avoid pitching with arm fatigue

3. Avoid excess pitching
   a. Follow published recommended pitch counts
   b. Do not pitch competitively more than 8 months a year

4. Monitor pitchers closely who
   a. Throw greater than 85 mph
   b. Are taller and heavier
   c. Are regularly starting pitchers
   d. Compete for multiple teams at once or pitch year round
   e. Participate in showcases

be performed to assess for a symptomatic posteromedial olecranon osteophyte, which may need to be excised at the time of UCL reconstruction. This is done by passively snapping the elbow into extension while maintaining valgus stress at the elbow. Posterior medial elbow pain indicates a positive test. Neurovascular examination should be performed looking specifically for evidence of ulnar nerve dysfunction. Most commonly this is elicited as a positive Tinel test at the cubital tunnel (21%[1]); however, more significant dysfunction, including hand intrinsic muscle weakness and wasting can be present and should be looked for and documented. Finally, the remainder of the upper extremity needs to be evaluated, including assessment of ROM and strength at the shoulder, elbow, and wrist. It is not uncommon for shoulder and elbow pathology to coexist and failure to address both can be detrimental to any treatment on the elbow.

Radiographic evaluation is completed in all patients with concern for UCL injury. Standard radiographs of the elbow, including anteroposterior, medial and lateral oblique, axial olecranon, and lateral views are obtained to evaluate bony abnormalities. Fifty-seven percent of patients will show some abnormality; most commonly olecranon osteophyte formation or ectopic calcification within the UCL substance.[1] Stress radiography with valgus stress on the elbow can be obtained, but has been found to rarely change the treatment course. In addition, the views can be somewhat difficult to interpret, as there is often an increased medial elbow opening in the dominant arm of uninjured throwing athletes compared with their nondominant side.[13] In any athlete with concern for UCL tear after examination and radiographs, magnetic resonance (MR) arthrogram of the elbow should be obtained. Partial undersurface tears of the UCL are common, and a contrasted study can better visualize these. The T-sign (**Fig. 5**) was originally described by Timmerman and colleagues[14] using computed tomography (CT) arthrography, and describes the pattern of contrast tracking with partial undersurface detachment of the UCL. Although this was initially described using CT, MR arthrography is now considered the gold standard given its superior ability to evaluate soft tissue structures. Using MR arthrogram, Schwartz and colleagues[15]

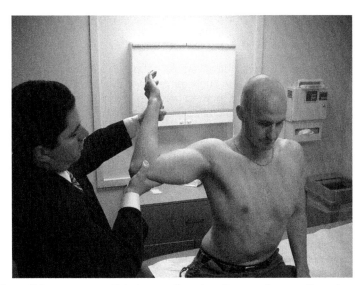

Fig. 4. The milking maneuver. Pain is reproduced as the examiner applies valgus stress by pulling the thumb with the elbow in the throwing position.

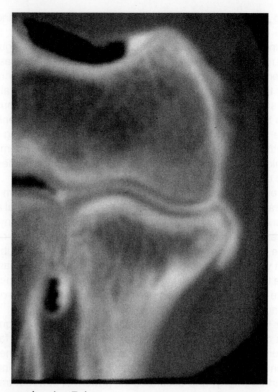

Fig. 5. CT arthrogram showing T-sign.

were able to detect UCL tears correctly in 93% of patients, including 86% of partial tears. In studies of noncontrasted MRI for UCL injury, partial tears were identified only 14% of the time.[14]

NONOPERATIVE MANAGEMENT

The decision to proceed with operative versus nonoperative treatment is largely based on informed decision making between the athlete and doctor; however, nonoperative treatment is recommended for 3 months before performing reconstruction. Due to season-specific schedules and time-sensitive demands in high-level throwers, operative treatment is often chosen without an extended period of conservative treatment. Nonoperative treatment consists of complete rest from throwing for at least 3 months as well as avoiding any activities that place valgus stress across the elbow. Rehabilitation is initiated immediately for both the elbow and shoulder. At the 3-month mark, if all symptoms in the elbow have resolved, an interval throwing program is initiated. The athlete is progressed through the throwing program as tolerated and gradually returned to sport after the throwing program is completed (further details regarding the throwing program are provided later in this article).

Rettig and colleagues[16] followed a group of 31 overhead throwing athletes with UCL injuries that elected for nonoperative treatment. They found that 13 (42%) were able to return to their sport at an average of 24.5 weeks. No predictive findings, obtained either through the patient's history or physical examination, were identified that would assist the clinician or athlete in predicting the success of nonoperative treatment.

As the role of biologics in orthopedics continues to be explored, there is hope that local biological enhancement of UCL injuries may expand our options for nonoperative treatment. Currently there is only 1 study evaluating their use. Podesta and colleagues[17] injected type 1A platelet-rich plasma (PRP) (leukocyte-rich, unactivated, $5\times$ or > platelet concentration[18]) into 34 elbows (27 baseball players) with MRI-confirmed partial UCL tears. The athletes then underwent a rehabilitation program, which strictly limited stress across the UCL. Athletes were allowed to return to sport based on symptoms and examination findings. Eighty-eight percent returned to the same level of play without complaints an average of 12 weeks after injection.[17] Given these initial results, further evaluation of PRP and other orthobiologics is certainly warranted to expand our nonoperative treatment options.

OPERATIVE MANAGEMENT

Multiple operative techniques have been described for UCL reconstruction. At our institution, UCL reconstruction is performed with the modified Jobe technique as described by Azar and colleagues.[19] Arthroscopy before reconstruction was routinely performed at our institution until we recognized that arthroscopy rarely changed the preoperative plan.[1] Currently, the presence of anterior pathology, such as loose bodies or osteochondral defect, is our only indication for arthroscopy before reconstruction.

Ipsilateral palmaris autograft is our current graft of choice. This must be examined preoperatively because 16% of patients have unilateral absence and 9% have bilateral absence.[20] In revision cases or in patients with insufficient or absent palmaris, contralateral gracilis tendon followed by contralateral palmaris is used. The contralateral gracilis is chosen because of ease of setup and position of the surgeon during the harvest. Gracilis tendon is also our first choice in cases with bony involvement of the ligament in which there is not sufficient native ligament to repair to the graft.[21] Toe extensors, plantaris, and patellar tendon grafts also have been used. One recent study showed that graft choice and diameter of graft had no effect on resistance to valgus stress, and that all reconstruction types restored valgus resistance at 60 to 120° of flexion.[22]

In our technique, the patient is positioned supine with an arm board for the operative extremity. If the gracilis tendon is chosen, the contralateral leg is prepped and draped simultaneously. A tourniquet is inflated after exsanguination of the extremity. A medial approach is performed, and the medial antebrachial nerve is located and protected. The ulnar nerve is then located in the cubital tunnel and mobilized. Ulnar nerve transposition is performed in all cases regardless of the presence of nerve symptoms preoperatively. Transposition of the ulnar nerve is necessary to allow elevation of the deep flexor muscle mass and UCL exposure when using the modified Jobe technique. The ulnar nerve neurolysis extends to the deep portion of the flexor carpi ulnaris distally and proximally to the Arcade of Struthers. Once the decompression is complete, the nerve is retracted with a vessel loop (**Fig. 6**). The flexor muscle mass is not released from the medial epicondyle, rather it is elevated and retracted anteriorly by small Hohmann retractors. The UCL is identified beneath the flexor muscle mass, as are its attachments to the medial epicondyle and sublime tubercle (**Fig. 7**). If no tear is seen on the superficial surface of the ligament, a longitudinal incision is made through the ligament. Undersurface tears, partial tears, and avulsions can then be identified. Any portion of the ligament that is degenerative should be excised, leaving only healthy-appearing ligament.

The autologous graft of choice is then harvested. Our technique for palmaris harvest is performed with three 1-cm transverse incisions. The palmaris is palpated and

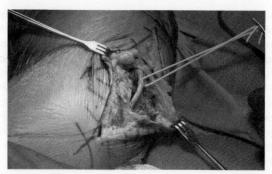

Fig. 6. The ulnar nerve is dissected free from the cubital tunnel and mobilized with a vessel loop.

marked with the first incision made near the distal wrist crease, and the second incision is made 3 to 4 cm proximal to the first. The tendon is found in both distal incisions and cut distally with the wrist flexed to maximize tendon length. The tendon is then pulled through the second incision and tensioned to identify the most proximal location the tendon can be palpated. A third incision is made directly over this point and carried down to cut the tendon (**Fig. 8**). This usually provides a graft length of 15 to 20 cm; 13 cm is the minimum graft length to ensure good graft fixation. Muscle is removed from the tendon and each end is secured with a No. 1 nonabsorbable suture in locking fashion.

If posterior osteophytes are present, they are removed through a posterior, vertical arthrotomy. Over-resection of the olecranon must be avoided, as this can further destabilize the elbow and place increased stress on the reconstruction. Posterior loose bodies, if present, also can be removed through this arthrotomy at this time.

Tunnel placement is absolutely critical to surgical success. Two convergent tunnels are drilled at the origin site of the UCL in the medial epicondyle (**Fig. 9**) in a Y fashion and 2 convergent tunnels are drilled at the insertion site of the sublime tubercle in a U or V fashion. A 3.2-mm drill bit is used with palmaris grafts and a 4.0-mm drill bit is used with gracilis tendon grafts. After drilling the first tunnel on each side, a hemostat is placed in the tunnel as an aiming point to ensure a complete tunnel is made. Graft passage begins on the ulnar side and a bent Hewson suture passer is used to pass one end of the graft through the ulna (**Fig. 10**). The native ligament is next repaired

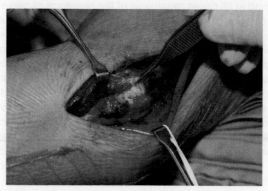

Fig. 7. The flexor digitorum profundus muscle belly is elevated to expose the native ulnar collateral ligament.

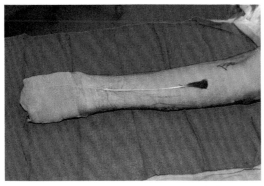

Fig. 8. The palmaris graft is confirmed at all 3 incision sites before it is cut distally, secured with a whipstitch, and delivered out of the proximal wound.

while it is still easily accessible. Next, the 2 limbs of the tendon graft are passed through the humeral tunnels creating a figure-of-8 (**Fig. 11**). A varus stress is applied with the elbow at roughly 30° and the 2 limbs are tied together with No. 1 nonabsorbable suture. The 2 limbs are then tied side-to-side at the level of the joint incorporating the native ligament to add increased soft tissue strength to the reconstruction (**Fig. 12**).

The subcutaneous ulnar nerve transposition is performed using a strip of medial intermuscular septum. This is left intact to its insertion at the medial epicondyle and the free end is sewn to the flexor-pronator muscle fascia with 3 to 0 nonabsorbable suture creating a sling for the ulnar nerve. Enough length should be harvested from the septum to ensure there is no compression on the nerve. Closure of the flexor carpi ulnaris fascial splint is important to prevent late propagation of the split that can lead to a fascial hernia. The deep posterior fascial tissue is also sewn to the periosteum of the medial epicondyle to further prevent subluxation of the nerve back into the groove. The skin is then closed in layered fashion over a superficial drain. The patient is placed in a well-padded posterior splint for 1 week, then the rehabilitation protocol is initiated as discussed later in this article.

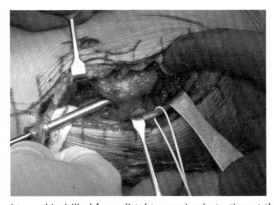

Fig. 9. The humeral tunnel is drilled from distal to proximal, starting at the native insertion of the ulnar collateral ligament onto the humerus.

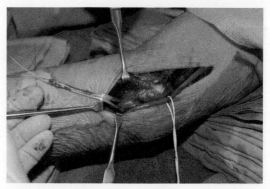

Fig. 10. The graft is passed through the ulnar tunnel.

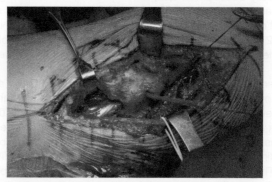

Fig. 11. The graft is passed through the humeral tunnels in a crossed, figure-of-8 manner (the anterior graft limb is passed through the more medial humeral tunnel).

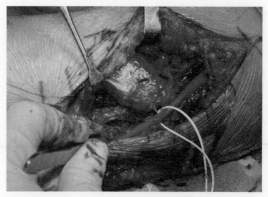

Fig. 12. The graft is sewn to the native UCL between the humeral and ulnar tunnels to increase tension within the graft and re-create the course of the native ligament.

There are multiple described alternatives to the modified Jobe technique. The docking technique described by Rohrbough and colleagues[23] uses a muscle-splitting approach without ulnar nerve transposition. A single Y-shaped humeral tunnel is made, and smaller proximal exit holes are made with a 1.5-mm drill bit. Rather than pass the graft out 2 proximal drill holes, the proximal ends are docked in the humerus, and the suture itself is tied over a humeral bone bridge (**Fig. 13**). These modifications were made due to concerns with the Jobe technique, specifically the ability to adequately tension the graft, the strength of the suture repair, the potential for complications due to detachment of the flexor origin, the creation of 2 large drill holes on the epicondyle, and excessive handling of the ulnar nerve.[23]

The David Altchek and Neal ElAttrache for Tommy John (DANE TJ) procedure is another commonly used approach to reconstruction.[24] This technique uses a combination of fixation techniques. On the humeral side, docking fixation is used to take advantage of smaller proximal drill holes. On the ulnar side, interference screw fixation is performed, with a single drill hole made at the UCL insertion site. The use of the single ulnar tunnel, in theory, decreases the risk of bony fracture and reduces the amount of surgical dissection required for exposure compared with the 2-tunnel technique. This technique also may be useful when the sublime tubercle is insufficient to provide an acceptable ulnar bone bridge, as may occur in revision situations or with sublime tubercle stress fracture.

POSTOPERATIVE REHABILITATION PROTOCOL

A standardized postoperative 4-phase rehabilitation program for ulnar collateral reconstruction as described by Wilk and colleagues is followed.[25–27] The first phase begins 1 week after surgery when the posterior splint placed at surgery is removed. The goals of phase I are to gradually restore full ROM at the elbow, decrease inflammation and pain, prevent muscular atrophy, and protect the healing UCL tissue. The shoulder, scapula, wrist, fingers, legs, and core are all emphasized during this time period while activities are limited at the elbow. The goal is for full ROM of the elbow joint to be restored by the end of the fifth to sixth week after surgery.

During phase II (weeks 9–12), a progressive isotonic strengthening program is initiated. Exercises continue to be focused on scapular, rotator cuff, deltoid, arm

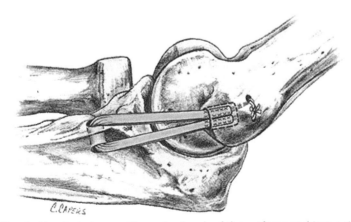

C.CAPERS

Fig. 13. The docking technique, with proximal ends of the graft secured into a single bone tunnel and sutures tied over a bone bridge.

musculature, legs, and core. Shoulder ROM and stretching exercises are performed during this phase and the Thrower's Ten Exercise Program is initiated. Any adaptations or strength deficits are addressed during this phase.

During the advanced strengthening phase (phase III), from weeks 13 to 16, a sport-specific exercise/rehabilitation program is initiated. Stretching and flexibility exercises are emphasized to enhance strength, power, and endurance. Isotonic strengthening exercises are progressed and the advanced Thrower's Ten Program is initiated. The athlete is allowed to begin an isotonic lifting program, including bench press, seated rowing, latissimus dorsi pull downs, triceps push downs, and biceps curls. A plyometric throwing program is begun at this point and the patient is progressed from 2-handed exercises to single-handed exercises.

Phase IV, the return to activity phase (week 16 and beyond), is characterized by the initiation of an interval throwing program. The criteria to return to throwing includes full nonpainful elbow ROM, elbow stability, satisfactory isokinetic test, and no pain with valgus stress, milking maneuver, or moving valgus stress test. Continued strengthening and stretching with persistent use of the Throwers Ten program and plyometric exercises is essential to protecting the elbow as the throwing program is progressed. All patients are counseled that there is no set time table for progressing through the throwing program and progressing faster than their body allows will increase their chance for reinjury (**Box 2**).

Our throwing program (for baseball athletes) consists of 2 phases. The first phase is for all position types and the patient is progressed from 45 feet to 180 feet over 6 stages (**Table 1**). Each stage requires the thrower to throw 75 times at a specified distance before advancing to the next stage. If an athlete has increased pain, the throwing program should be backed off and readvanced as tolerated. The throwing program should be performed every-other day, but can be spread out further if

---

Box 2
Standard 4 phase rehabilitation protocol for ulnar collateral ligament (UCL) reconstruction

UCL Reconstruction Rehabilitation

- Phase 1:
  - Gradually restore full range of motion (ROM) at the elbow
  - Decrease inflammation and pain
  - Prevent muscular atrophy
  - Protect the healing UCL tissue
  - The shoulder, scapula, wrist, fingers, legs, and core are all emphasized

- Phase 2:
  - Isotonic strengthening begins
  - Continue shoulder ROM and stretching exercises
  - Thrower's Ten Exercise Program is initiated
  - Any adaptations or strength deficits are addressed during this phase

- Phase 3:
  - Sports-specific strengthening and rehabilitation is initiated
  - Advanced Thrower's Ten Program is begun
  - Stretching and flexibility is emphasized
  - Isotonic lifting program should include bench press, triceps push downs, and biceps curls
  - A plyometric throwing program is progressed from 2-handed exercises to single-handed exercises

- Phase 4:
  - Continued strengthening, stretching, Thrower's Ten Program, and plyometric exercises
  - Initiation of interval throwing program

Table 1
Phase I (flat ground) interval throwing program

45' Phase	60' Phase	90' Phase	120' Phase

Step 1:
A. Warm-up throwing
B. 45' (25 throws)
C. Rest 5–10 min
D. Warm-up throwing
E. 45' (25 throws)
 	
Step 2:
A. Warm-up throwing
B. 45' (25 throws)
C. Rest 5–10 min
D. Warm-up throwing
E. 45' (25 throws)
F. Rest 5–10 min
G. Warm-up throwing
H. 45' (25 throws)
	Step 3:
	A. Warm-up
	    throwing
	B. 60' (25 throws)
	C. Rest 5–10 min
	D. Warm-up
	    throwing
	E. 60' (25 throws)
	
	Step 4:
	A. Warm-up
	    throwing
	B. 60' (25 throws)
	C. Rest 5–10 min
	D. Warm-up
	    throwing
	E. 60' (25 throws)
	F. Rest 5–10 min
	G. Warm-up
	    throwing
	H. 60' (25 throws)
		Step 5:
		A. Warm-up
		    throwing
		B. 90' (25 throws)
		C. Rest 5–10 min
		D. Warm-up
		    throwing
		E. 90' (25 throws)
		
		Step 6:
		A. Warm-up
		    throwing
		B. 90' (25 throws)
		C. Rest 5–10 min
		D. Warm-up
		    throwing
		E. 90' (25 throws)
		F. Rest 5–10 min
		G. Warm-up
		    throwing
		H. 90' (25 throws)
			Step 7:
			A. Warm-up throwing
			B. 120' (25 throws)
			C. Rest 5–10 min
			D. Warm-up throwing
			E. 120' (25 throws)
			
			Step 8:
			A. Warm-up throwing
			B. 120' (25 throws)
			C. Rest 5–10 min
			D. Warm-up throwing
			E. 120' (25 throws)
			F. Rest 5–10 min
			G. Warm-up throwing
			H. 120' (25 throws)

150' Phase	180' Phase		

Step 9:
A. Warm-up throwing
B. 150' (25 throws)
C. Rest 5–10 min
D. Warm-up throwing
E. 150' (25 throws)
 	
Step 10:
A. Warm-up throwing
B. 150' (25 throws)
C. Rest 5–10 min
D. Warm-up throwing
E. 150' (25 throws)
F. Rest 5–10 min
G. Warm-up throwing
H. 150' (25 throws)
	Step 11:
	A. Warm-up
	    throwing
	B. 180' (25 throws)
	C. Rest 5–10 min
	D. Warm-up
	    throwing
	E. 180' (25 throws)
	
	Step 12:
	A. Warm-up
	    throwing
	B. 180' (25 throws)
	C. Rest 5–10 min
	D. Warm-up
	    throwing
	E. 180' (25 throws)
	F. Rest 5–10 min
	G. Warm-up
	    throwing
	H. 180' (25 throws)
		Step 13:
		A. Warm-up
		    throwing
		B. 180' (25 throws)
		C. Rest 5–10 min
		D. Warm-up
		    throwing
		E. 180' (25 throws)
		
		Step 14:
		Begin throwing
		    off the mound
		    or return to
		    respective
		    position.
			Throwing program
			    should be
			    performed every-
			    other day, unless
			    otherwise specified
			    by your physician or
			    rehabilitation
			    specialist.
			Perform each step __
			    times before
			    progressing to next
			    step.

Flat Ground Throwing

A. Warm-up throwing
B. Throw 60' (10–15 throws)
C. Throw 90' (10 throws)
D. Throw 120' (10 throws)
E. Throw 60' (flat ground) using
    pitching mechanics (20–30 throws)

more time is needed to recover between throwing sessions. After all stages have been completed, position players can begin throwing in simulated game-type situations progressing from 50% to 75% to 100% effort as they feel comfortable and without pain. Pitchers should move on to phase II, which progresses them throwing off the mound. Pitchers begin with fastballs only and gradually increase in the number and intensity of pitches. Off speed and breaking ball type pitches are added once full effort with fastball pitches has been achieved. Phase II ends with the beginning of simulated game pitching (**Box 3**). Pitchers start with a 15-throw pitch count and can progress by 10 throws each outing. Although there is no set speed that can or should progress through these phases, a gradual return to competition can be expected for pitchers at approximately 10 to 12 months and position players at 6 to 7 months postoperative.

OUTCOMES/RETURN TO OVERHAND THROWING

Results after UCL reconstruction have overall been quite good. In the largest single series of UCL reconstruction reported to date, Cain and colleagues[1] followed 743 patients (95% baseball players, 89% pitchers) after UCL reconstruction with a mean follow-up time of 49.1 months; 83% of athletes in their study were able to return to sports at the same or higher as compared with preinjury.[1] Recently, Osbahr and colleagues[28] published a 10-year follow-up on the same cohort of patients. In total, they

---

Box 3
Phase II (mound) interval throwing program

Stage 1: Fastballs only

Step 1: Interval throwing - 15 throws off mound 50% (use interval throwing to 120′ phase as warm-up)

Step 2: Interval throwing - 30 throws off mound 50%

Step 3: Interval throwing - 45 throws off mound 50% (all throwing off the mound should be done in the presence of your pitching coach to stress proper throwing mechanics)

Step 4: Interval throwing - 60 throws off mound 50%

Step 5: Interval throwing - 70 throws off mound 50% (use speed gun to aid in effort control)

Step 6: 45 throws off mound 50%; 30 throws off mound 75%

Step 7: 30 throws off mound 50%; 45 throws off mound 75%

Step 8: 65 throws off mound 75%; 10 throws off mound 50%

Stage 2: Fastballs only

Step 9: 60 throws off mound 75%; 15 throws in batting practice

Step 10: 50 to 60 throws off mound 75%; 30 throws in batting practice

Step 11: 45 to 50 throws off mound 75%; 45 throws in batting practice

Stage 3

Step 12: 30 throws off mound 75% warm-up; 15 throws off mound 50% breaking balls; 45 to 60 throws in batting practice (fastball only)

Step 13: 30 throws off mound 75%; 30 breaking balls 75%; 30 throws in batting practice

Step 14: 30 throws off mound 75%; 60 to 90 throws in batting practice (gradually increase breaking balls)

Step 15: Simulated game - progressing by 15 throws per workout (pitch count)

had follow-up on 256 patients at average of 12.6 years. They found that career longevity after UCL reconstruction was 3.6 years, and only 2.9 years at a level that was equal or higher to preinjury. Interestingly, they found retirement from baseball due to reasons other than elbow problems in 86% of respondents and that subsequent shoulder problems were the most commonly cited reason for retirement. Overall, 93% of patients were satisfied with the operation and 98% were still able to throw at least on a recreational level.

In 2008, Vitale and Ahmad[29] published a systematic review of the outcomes of UCL reconstruction in overhead athletes. In total, this included 7 studies with 405 patients. They similarly found 83% excellent outcomes with studies published later having improved outcomes to those published earlier in the literature. They also analyzed variables related to surgical technique and found that techniques that involved a muscle-splitting approach to the flexor-pronator mass had a higher percentage of excellent outcomes (87%) compared with retraction (81%) or detachment (70%) of the flexor-pronator mass. Graft fixation technique showed a difference in results as well. Figure-of-8 technique had a 76% excellent result compared with 90% for docking and 95% for modified docking (consisting of tripling of the graft).

A more recent systematic review including 20 studies was performed by Erickson and colleagues.[30] They showed an overall 82% excellent and 8% good outcomes with 86.2% return to play. The docking technique had the highest rate of return to play (97%) compared with the modified Jobe technique (93%) and the Jobe technique (66%). Collegiate athletes had the highest return to sport (95%) compared with high school athletes (89%) and professional athletes (86%).

In a study looking at pitchers at the major league level only, Mekhni and colleagues[31] reviewed 147 pitchers who underwent UCL reconstruction. They found 80% of these pitchers were able to return to pitch in at least 1 game, whereas only 67% were able to return to an established level, which they defined as pitching more than 10 outings in a season. They also found that disabled list visits after UCL reconstruction for elbow-related issues were significantly lower than before surgery. In a similar study looking at only professional baseball pitchers, Erikson and colleagues[32] followed 179 pitchers after undergoing UCL reconstruction; 83% were able to return to play at the Major League Baseball (MLB) level and 97.2% returned to either the major or minor leagues. The average length of career after return from UCL surgery was 3.9 years.

The time to return to play after UCL reconstruction has varied widely across the literature. Cain and colleagues[1] reported an average return to play after 11.6 months compared with 20.5 months in the review by Erikson and colleagues[32] of MLB pitchers. Makhni and colleagues,[31] Gibson and colleagues,[33] and Koh and colleagues[34] had average return to play of 16.8, 18.5, and 13.1 months, respectively. The wide array of reported time to return to play highlights the diversity of rehabilitation protocols that are followed after surgery and the lack of a uniformly accepted approach to rehabilitation. The minimal amount of time and rehabilitation of the elbow and shoulder required to safely return to overhead throwing after UCL reconstruction is still yet to be determined based on our current literature. Further research on this area is certainly warranted.

Several studies have looked to quantify how well athletes, in particular pitchers, return to their sport after UCL surgery. Overall, the objective results after UCL reconstruction have been quite good. Fleisig and colleagues[35] looked at the biomechanical performance of minor league baseball pitchers who had undergone UCL reconstruction and compared them to a matched control group with no history of injury to their shoulder or elbow. They found there was no difference in pitching biomechanics between the 2 groups. This group did reflect only those athletes who were able to make it back to a minor league level of competition, however, and the data may be different if those who were unable to return had been included as well.

Makhani and colleagues[31] collected performance data in multiple statistical categories on 92 MLB pitchers for up to 3 years before and after UCL reconstruction surgery. When comparing preinjury to postsurgery performance, they found that the statistical measures declined in virtually all recorded categories; however, when these declines were compared with a cohort of 192 aged-matched healthy controls they found this group underwent similar regressions in statistical measures with age. Erickson and colleagues[32] looked at a similar group of MLB pitchers who underwent UCL reconstruction and compared them to a matched control group. They found that pitchers who had undergone UCL reconstruction had a lower earned run average and walks plus hits per inning pitched than before surgery and also when compared with the control group.

The effect of UCL reconstruction on velocity has been evaluated in a couple of different studies. Lansdown and Feeley[36] looked specifically at the pitch velocity of 80 MLB pitchers after UCL reconstruction using publicly available data. They found that mean fastball velocity was significantly decreased following surgery, falling from a presurgery mean of 91.3 mph to a postoperative velocity of 90.6 mph. This effect was most notably pronounced in pitchers older than 35 in whom the preinjury to postoperative change was 2.9 mph. Interestingly, pitch velocity for other commonly thrown pitches such as curveballs, changeups, and sliders did not significantly decline. Jiang and Leland[37] also evaluated pitch velocity in a group of MLB pitchers who underwent UCL reconstruction. In addition, they compared them to a pair-matched control group of pitchers without known UCL injury. They similarly found a small but statistically significant decrease in velocity in the postsurgical years; however, when compared with the control group, there was no difference at any time point or for any type of pitch. Makhani and colleagues[31] reviewed performance data in MLB pitchers and had similar findings of decreased velocity after surgery but no greater decline than age-matched uninjured controls.

Previous studies demonstrate that revision UCL reconstruction is a relatively uncommon procedure. In the series by Cain and colleagues[1] of 743 patients, only 9 (1%) athletes required a revision reconstruction. Similarly, in the systematic review performed by Erikson and colleagues,[30] the revision rate was noted to be 0.7%. As the number of primary UCL reconstructions continues to grow, it would be expected that so too would the number of revision UCL reconstructions. Unfortunately, there is only sparse outcomes data on athletes' function after revision UCL surgery. Dines and colleagues[38] performed a retrospective review on 15 baseball players who underwent revision UCL reconstruction and found that only 33% were able to return to their preinjury level of competition. They noted a much higher return rate in MLB players (75%) compared with minor league players (14%). Jones and colleagues[39] performed the largest review of functional outcomes after revision UCL reconstruction. They retrospectively identified 18 MLB pitchers who had revision UCL reconstruction between 1996 and 2009 and found that 78% of pitchers were able to return to the major league level within 2 full seasons of their surgery. Postsurgery workload, however, was significantly decreased in this population, with relief pitchers regaining only about 50% and starting pitchers 35% of their preinjury pitch workload.

The most frequent complication after UCL surgery is transient ulnar neuritis, which accounts for 75% of all postoperative complications and occurs in approximately 7.9% of patients.[30] Donor site issues, including pain, wound dehiscence, weakness, and paresthesia are the next most common complaints, accounting for approximately

13% of all complications.[30] Major complications, including ulnar tunnel fracture (0.1%) or need for subsequent elbow surgery (5%), are infrequent occurrences. The most common reason for subsequent elbow surgery is for olecranon osteophyte excision.[1] In the revision UCL setting, the complication rate has been noted to be considerably higher (40%).[38]

SUMMARY

UCL injuries can be disabling in throwers. Reconstruction has afforded throwers a high rate of return to preinjury function, and several techniques have been presented that produce acceptable results. Overall complication rates are low, and most complications are transient ulnar neurapraxias. Increased involvement in youth sports and year-round participation is increasing injury rates in young athletes. The orthopedic community must continue to look for better ways to prevent these injuries and investigate better methods to return athletes to high-level competition.

REFERENCES

1. Cain EL, Andrews JR, Dugas JR, et al. Outcome of ulnar collateral ligament reconstruction of the elbow in 1281 athletes results in 743 athletes with minimum 2-year follow-up. Am J Sports Med 2010;38(12):2426–34.
2. Erickson BJ, Nwachukwu BU, Rosas S, et al. Trends in medial ulnar collateral ligament reconstruction in the United States: a retrospective review of a large private-payer database from 2007 to 2011. Am J Sports Med 2015;43(7):1770–4.
3. Fuss FK. The ulnar collateral ligament of the human elbow joint. Anatomy, function and biomechanics. J Anat 1991;175:203.
4. Floris S, Olsen BS, Dalstra M, et al. The medial collateral ligament of the elbow joint: anatomy and kinematics. J Shoulder Elbow Surg 1998;7(4):345–51.
5. Dugas JR, Ostrander RV, Cain EL, et al. Anatomy of the anterior bundle of the ulnar collateral ligament. J Shoulder Elbow Surg 2007;16(5):657–60.
6. Fleisig GS, Andrews JR, Dillman CJ. Kinetics of baseball pitching with implications about injury mechanism. Am J Sports Med 1995;23:233–9.
7. Morrey BF, An KN. Articular and ligamentous contributions to the stability of the elbow joint. Am J Sports Med 1983;11:315–9.
8. Fleisig GS, Andrews JR. Prevention of elbow injuries in youth baseball pitchers. Sports Health 2012;4(5):419–24.
9. Olsen SJ, Fleisig GS, Dun S, et al. Risk factors for shoulder and elbow injuries in adolescent baseball pitchers. Am J Sports Med 2006;34(6):905–12.
10. Zaremski JL, Horodyski M, Donlan RM, et al. Does geographic location matter on the prevalence of ulnar collateral ligament reconstruction in collegiate baseball pitchers? Orthop J Sports Med 2015;3(11). 2325967115616582.
11. Bruce JR, Andrews JR. Ulnar collateral ligament injuries in the throwing athlete. J Am Acad Orthop Surg 2014;22(5):315–25.
12. O'Driscoll SW, Lawton RL, Smith AM. The "moving valgus stress test" for medial collateral ligament tears of the elbow. Am J Sports Med 2005;33(2):231–9.
13. Ellenbecker TS, Mattalino AJ, Elam EA, et al. Medial elbow joint laxity in professional baseball pitchers: a bilateral comparison using stress radiography. Am J Sports Med 1998;26(3):420–4.
14. Timmerman LA, Schwartz ML, Andrews JR. Preoperative evaluation of the ulnar collateral ligament by magnetic resonance imaging and computed tomography arthrography evaluation in 25 baseball players with surgical confirmation. Am J Sports Med 1994;22(1):26–32.

15. Schwartz ML, Al-Zahrani S, Morwessel RM, et al. Ulnar collateral ligament injury in the throwing athlete: evaluation with saline-enhanced MR arthrography. Radiology 1995;197(1):297–9.

16. Rettig AC, Sherrill C, Snead DS, et al. Nonoperative treatment of ulnar collateral ligament injuries in throwing athletes. Am J Sports Med 2001;29(1):15–7.

17. Podesta L, Crow SA, Volkmer D, et al. Treatment of partial ulnar collateral ligament tears in the elbow with platelet-rich plasma. Am J Sports Med 2013;41(7): 1689–94.

18. Mishra A, Harmon K, Woodall J, et al. Sports medicine applications of platelet rich plasma. Curr Pharm Biotechnol 2012;13(7):1185–95.

19. Azar FM, Andrews JR, Wilk KE, et al. Operative treatment of ulnar collateral ligament injuries of the elbow in athletes. Am J Sports Med 2000;28(1):16–23.

20. Thompson NW, Mockford BJ, Cran GW. Absence of the palmaris longus muscle: a population study. Ulster Med J 2001;70(1):22.

21. Dugas JR, Bilotta J, Watts CD, et al. Ulnar collateral ligament reconstruction with gracilis tendon in athletes with intraligamentous bony excision technique and results. Am J Sports Med 2012;40(7):1578–82.

22. Dargel J, Küpper F, Wegmann K, et al. Graft diameter does not influence primary stability of ulnar collateral ligament reconstruction of the elbow. J Orthop Sci 2015;20(2):307–13.

23. Rohrbough JT, Altchek DW, Hyman J, et al. Medial collateral ligament reconstruction of the elbow using the docking technique. Am J Sports Med 2002;30(4): 541–8.

24. Conway JE. The DANE TJ procedure for elbow medial ulnar collateral ligament insufficiency. Tech Shoulder Elbow Surg 2006;7(1):36–43.

25. Wilk KE, Arrigo CA, Andrews JR. Rehabilitation of the elbow in the throwing athlete. J Orthop Sports Phys Ther 1993;17:305–17.

26. Wilk KE, Arrigo CA, Andrews JR, et al. Rehabilitation following elbow surgery in the throwing athlete. Oper Tech Sports Med 1996;4:114–32.

27. Wilk KE, Arrigo CA, Andrews JR, et al. Preventative and rehabilitation exercises for the shoulder and elbow. 4th edition. Birmingham (AL): American Sports Medicine Institute; 1996.

28. Osbahr DC, Cain EL, Raines BT, et al. Long-term outcomes after ulnar collateral ligament reconstruction in competitive baseball players: minimum 10-year follow-up. Am J Sports Med 2014;42(6):1333–42.

29. Vitale MA, Ahmad CS. The outcome of elbow ulnar collateral ligament reconstruction in overhead athletes: a systematic review. Am J Sports Med 2008;36(6): 1193–205.

30. Erickson BJ, Chalmers PN, Bush-Joseph CA, et al. Ulnar collateral ligament reconstruction of the elbow: a systematic review of the literature. Orthop J Sports Med 2015;3(12). 2325967115618914.

31. Makhni EC, Lee RW, Morrow ZS, et al. Performance, return to competition, and reinjury after Tommy John surgery in major league baseball pitchers: a review of 147 cases. Am J Sports Med 2014;42(6):1323–32.

32. Erickson BJ, Gupta AK, Harris JD, et al. Rate of return to pitching and performance after Tommy John surgery in Major League Baseball pitchers. Am J Sports Med 2014;42(3):536–43.

33. Gibson BW, Webner D, Huffman GR, et al. Ulnar collateral ligament reconstruction in major league baseball pitchers. Am J Sports Med 2007;35(4):575–81.

34. Koh JL, Schafer MF, Keuter G, et al. Ulnar collateral ligament reconstruction in elite throwing athletes. Arthroscopy 2006;22(11):1187–91.

35. Fleisig GS, Leddon CE, Laughlin WA, et al. Biomechanical performance of base-ball pitchers with a history of ulnar collateral ligament reconstruction. Am J Sports Med 2015;43(5):1045–50.
36. Lansdown DA, Feeley BT. The effect of ulnar collateral ligament reconstruction on pitch velocity in Major League Baseball pitchers. Orthop J Sports Med 2014;2(2). 2325967114522592.
37. Jiang JJ, Leland JM. Analysis of pitching velocity in major league baseball players before and after ulnar collateral ligament reconstruction. Am J Sports Med 2014;42(4):880–5.
38. Dines JS, Yocum LA, Frank JB, et al. Revision surgery for failed elbow medial collateral ligament reconstruction. Am J Sports Med 2008;36(6):1061–5.
39. Jones KJ, Conte S, Patterson N, et al. Functional outcomes following revision ul-nar collateral ligament reconstruction in Major League Baseball pitchers. J Shoulder Elbow Surg 2013;22(5):642–6.

Return to Play After Hand and Wrist Fractures

Andrea Halim, MD, Arnold-Peter C. Weiss, MD*

KEYWORDS

- Carpal fractures • Hand fractures • Scaphoid fractures • Return to play

KEY POINTS

- Return to play can be initiated safely after many hand and wrist injuries with playing casts or other protective gear.
- Early diagnosis and appropriate treatment can allow athletes to return to play quickly after they sustain fractures or dislocations of the hand or wrist.
- The treating surgeon should weigh the athlete's needs and level of competition with likelihood of reinjury when counseling on return to play guidelines.

INTRODUCTION

For athletes playing contact sports or ball sports, manual dexterity and normal hand biomechanics are crucial to success. Hand and wrist injuries in these athletes may leave them permanently disadvantaged in their sport, if inadequately treated. One of the orthopedist's goals is to allow the player to return to their sport in a timely fashion, but with minimal risk for long-term disability.

Hand and wrist injuries are encountered frequently in athletes, and make up 3% to 9% of athletic injuries.[1] Football is the most common sport leading to hand and wrist injury.[2] For the professional or elite college athlete, rapid return to sport may be the priority for the patient and surgeon. Management priorities may be different for recreational or younger athletes, when long-term function and healing with minimal risk of complication are the primary considerations. These principles may have a strong effect on treatment decisions, and may also be reflected in the surgeon's approach to return to play.

One of the tools in the surgeon's armamentarium is the playing cast. The availability and application of immobilization that is safe for an athlete to wear during play can often allow them to return to their sport before complete healing. A variety of playing

Division of Hand Surgery, Department of Orthopaedics, Alpert Medical School of Brown University, 2 Dudley Street, Suite 200, Providence, RI 02905, USA
* Corresponding author.
E-mail address: arnold-peter_weiss@brown.edu

Clin Sports Med 35 (2016) 597–608
http://dx.doi.org/10.1016/j.csm.2016.05.005   **sportsmed.theclinics.com**
0278-5919/16/$ – see front matter © 2016 Elsevier Inc. All rights reserved.

casts have been designed. In select scenarios, as discussed in further detail, these casts can allow athletes to safely return to sport.

DISTAL RADIUS FRACTURES

Distal radius fractures are among the most common injuries treated by orthopedic surgeons. However, less than 10% of these occur as a result of athletic injury.[3] They occur as a wide spectrum of disease, ranging from minimally displaced extraarticular fractures to high-energy fractures with articular comminution. The particular fracture pattern and characteristics determine the surgeon's approach to fracture management for the injured athlete.

Nonoperative Management

Nonoperative management is often selected for patients who demonstrate the following characteristics:

- Articular congruity without less than 2 mm stepoff
- Extraarticular simple fractures
- Radial height of at least 10 mm
- Radial inclination 22°
- Neutral volar tilt

However, even in cases in which nonoperative treatment is warranted, athletes should anticipate 6 to 8 weeks of immobilization. Typically, immobilization consists of a period of above-the-elbow splinting or casting. For the athlete, this may preclude many sports, and may result in elbow stiffness. They should be counseled regarding this possibility. When the fracture pattern allows, transition to a short-arm cast may allow athletes to return to play with less inconvenience and improved mobility.

Operative Management

Distal radius fractures vary widely, as do surgical approaches. Operative management of distal radius fractures is often selected for intraarticular fractures or those with characteristics of instability. Surgical options can include open reduction with volar locked plating, dorsal bridge plates, fragment-specific plating, and interfocal pinning.

After operative intervention, cast immobilization or removable splinting is usually continued for a period of 4 to 6 weeks. When stability allows, patients may begin early range of motion exercises after internal fixation. Return to sport depends largely on the stability of the fracture as well as sport-specific wrist motion requirements. Noncontact athletes may return to sport quickly after internal fixation, whereas high-impact athletes should refrain from return to sport until there is clinical and radiographic evidence of healing.[4]

SCAPHOID FRACTURES

The scaphoid bone is the most commonly fractured bone of the carpus.[5] Unfortunately, the scaphoid is notorious for being poorly healing for a variety of reasons. Because of their poor vascularity, retrograde blood supply, and inherent instability, scaphoid fractures can be challenging to treat. For the athlete, it is important to confirm healing to enable an ongoing career in sport.

Scaphoid fractures present occasionally as occult injuries, not clearly visible on radiographs.[6–8] In cases in which athletes present with significant snuffbox tenderness and a scaphoid fracture is suspected, early advanced imaging is an appropriate decision. MRI is very sensitive to diagnose scaphoid fractures. Given that initiation of immobilization within 3 to 4 weeks of injury improves chances of uncomplicated healing, it is to the athlete's benefit to obtain MRI when injury is suspected. When MRI is negative, the athlete can safely return to play without a period of immobilization.[8] Further, the early detection of scaphoid fractures has been shown to be cost effective compared with serial radiographs and casting of suspected injuries.[9] As a physician treating athletes, it is crucial in these cases to advocate for the patient and obtain advanced imaging when appropriate.

Nonoperative Management

Acute, nondisplaced fractures of the scaphoid waist can be treated by cast immobilization with a high rate of union. Although traditional treatment algorithms included immobilization in long-arm casts, more recent data have suggested that short-arm casting is sufficient. Further, it has been suggested that thumb immobilization does not affect union rates.[10] Short arm cast immobilization is much less unwieldy for the patient, and may allow athletes to participate in sports in select cases.

The criteria for treating a scaphoid in a cast include nondisplaced, acute fractures of the scaphoid waist. With early identification and initiation of casting, there is a greater than 90% rate of union. However, this treatment entails 6 to 12 weeks of immobilization.

Return to play can be allowed for both contact and noncontact sports during immobilization. Most athletes can safely return to play 4 weeks after injury in a playing cast.[11] If patients have a significant motivation to return to sport immediately, this may also be attempted, but requires careful monitoring and frequent cast changes. A protocol was developed that used short arm casts for football players, with silastic braces applied intermittently for games as per safety guidelines. In a series of 14 patients treated in this way, 12 patients went on to union, with 1 nonunion occurring in a proximal pole fracture and 1 nonunion occurring after a delay in diagnosis.[12]

Operative Management

Although nonoperative management remains the mainstay of nondisplaced scaphoid fractures, operative management offers several advantages, particularly in the situation of an athlete desiring early return to play.

Relative indications for operative management
- Scaphoid nonunion
- Displacement of more than 1 mm
- Humpback deformity
- Proximal pole fractures

When none of these indications is met, an athlete may still request early operative treatment. It has been established that compression screw placement early in the course of a scaphoid fracture allows earlier time to union, and more reliable union rates (**Fig. 1**).[13]

After fixation of scaphoid fracture with a headless compression screw, return to play guidelines vary significantly depending on sport and position, ranging from 2 weeks in a playing cast for noncontact athletes and to up to 12 weeks with a computed tomography scan for wrestlers, gymnasts, and weight lifters.[14] The athlete's demands and particular sport must be considered before the physician offers advice regarding return to play.

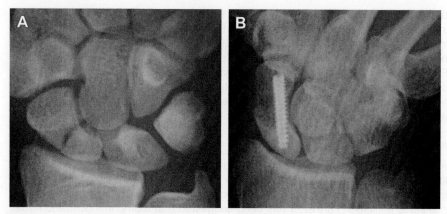

Fig. 1. A collegiate-level football player. (A) Anteroposterior radiograph of the wrist, demonstrating a scaphoid waist fracture. (B) Postoperative radiograph of the same patient. He was treated with a percutaneous compression screw, and returned to play immediately with instructions to wear a playing cast for 5 weeks.

OTHER CARPAL INJURIES

Hook of the Hamate Fractures

Hook of the hamate fractures are unusual injuries that can often be attributed to a strong blow against the base of the palm. Although they only make up 2% of carpal injuries, they can be seen in athletes who participate in racket sports, golf, and baseball.[15] These injuries can present significant morbidity, because they can affect the ulnar nerve and artery, or risk the flexor tendons to the ring and small fingers. They also present a significant risk for nonunion and ongoing pain during sport.

Patients with fractures of the hook of the hamate clinically present with ulnar-sided pain in the palm. They are best recognized either on plain radiographic carpal tunnel views or on computed tomography scan (**Fig. 2**). When recognized acutely, these fractures can be managed nonoperatively with casting. However, these injuries often present late, and with debilitating symptoms. In cases of nonunion, these fractures are best treated with simple excision.

After hook of hamate excision, athletes are typically immobilized for 2 to 3 weeks before initiation of therapy. Return to play after a hook of hamate excision is generally

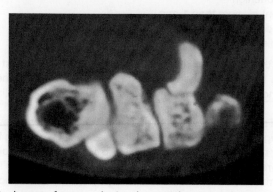

Fig. 2. Hook of the hamate fracture, depicted on axial computed tomography scan.

expected about 6 to 8 weeks after injury.[15,16] The palmar incision is sensitive for 4 to 6 weeks, and may benefit from desensitization before return to sport.[4] Athletes at the collegiate level can expect to have no change in sports performance compared with their baseline, and typically are satisfied with outcomes.[15]

Scapholunate Instability

Scapholunate ligament injury poses a challenging problem. These injuries occur most often with axial load on an extended wrist, and are seen frequently in football and other contact sports.[14,17] Scapholunate injuries sometimes present as static instability. These injuries demonstrate the "Terry Thomas sign," which is a widened scapholunate interval easily visible on radiographs (**Fig. 3**). However, some injuries present only with dynamic instability, and are diagnosed with the use of stress radiographs. These injuries may be treated with a period of cast immobilization, followed by return to play in playing casts.[17]

Acute, severe injuries may be treated by ligament repair and pinning. Ligament disruption often occurs from its insertion on the scaphoid, and repair of this injury may necessitate the use of suture anchors or bone tunnels. In these cases, repair may be augmented with capsulodesis or pinning.[17,18] In some cases, the scapholunate ligament may fail in its midsubstance. These injuries may be amenable to direct repair.

Chronic injuries pose an even more challenging problem. Several techniques have been developed in the setting of chronic scapholunate injury. These include tendon reconstruction with allograft or autograft, capsulodesis, and the use of compression screws. The Brunelli procedure involves passing a segment of the flexor carpi radialis through the scaphoid and securing it to the radius. The modification of this technique secures the flexor carpi radialis to the lunate or it's attachments, and avoids crossing the radiocarpal joint. After a modified Brunelli procedure, nearly 80% of professional athletes successfully return to sport within 4 months.[19]

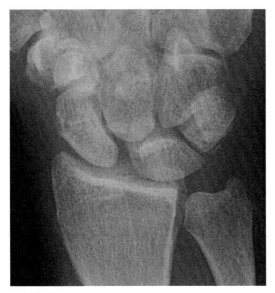

Fig. 3. Scapholunate widening is seen in this anteroposterior radiograph of the wrist, confirming an acute injury to the scapholunate ligament.

METACARPAL FRACTURES AND DISLOCATIONS
Metacarpal Fractures

Metacarpal fractures comprise a spectrum of injury, ranging from the benign boxer's fracture of the fifth metacarpal neck to multiple unstable shaft fractures. The majority of metacarpal fractures can be treated nonoperatively with return to sport after radiographic and clinical evidence of healing. However, a subset of these injuries represent significant risk for late dysfunction.

Metacarpal shaft

Closed, isolated fractures to the metacarpal shaft can be a result of a direct blow, a clenched fist injury, or a twisting injury. They are often amenable to closed reduction and immobilization. Athletes should be examined for concurrent injuries, and clinical and radiographic evaluation must be done to rule out significant shortening or malrotation.[4,20]

Athletes who sustain isolated metacarpal shaft fractures can be treated safely with immobilization and early return to play. If an athlete is eager to return to play and can tolerate it, a cast glove or similar hand-based immobilization technique can be used to facilitate wrist motion while protecting the fracture site.[21] Athletes can return to sport once circumferential callus is visible at the fracture site and there is clinical evidence of healing.[21]

Multiple metacarpal shaft fractures represent a more challenging problem, because this situation leads to inherent instability and the possibility of shortening. Reduction and fixation with K-wires, lag screws, or plates can offer stability and correct malalignment. For athletes, fixation with plates allows for early motion, and return to sport as soon as 2 weeks postoperatively, with 6 to 10 weeks of protection in a splint.[4]

Metacarpal neck

Injuries to the metacarpal neck are often seen as the result of closed-fist injuries, particularly at the fifth metacarpal. Fifth metacarpal neck fractures are generally well-tolerated owing to the relative mobility of the fourth and fifth carpometacarpal (CMC) joints.[4] These injuries can be treated typically by ulnar gutter cast immobilization with the interphalangeal joints left free. Some authors have successfully treated boxers' fracture with a soft wrap and buddy taping, with similar results.[22,23] Six weeks of immobilization is usually sufficient to ensure healing, and athletes can return to sport as early as pain and mobility allow.[4] Although patients may experience some loss of motion at the metacarpal–phalangeal joint, this typically has minimal clinical sequelae.[22]

Carpometacarpal Dislocations

Another commonly seen injury among athletes, particularly boxers, is the CMC dislocation. The fourth and fifth CMC joints are the most mobile, and the most prone to this injury. These injuries are easily missed on plain radiographs, so the orthopedic surgeon's suspicion should be high in the presence of significant dorsal hand swelling after an axial load. If CMC injury is suspected, a 30° pronated view often reveals the dislocation.[24]

Patients with dislocations of their fourth and fifth CMC joints can have good results if treated with closed reduction and immobilization alone.[25] However, patients with dislocations of the index or long finger metacarpal have a much higher risk of a poor outcome and continued pain.

Patients treated with reduction and stabilization of these injuries typically return to work within 3 months. Early management of these injuries also enable return to sport.[26] However, the risk of recurrent dislocation with axial loading makes this a challenging injury for which to counsel athletes, and should be done with caution.

PHALANX FRACTURES AND DISLOCATIONS
Proximal and Middle Phalanx Fractures

Fractures of the phalanges are relatively common injuries among athletes, especially for those who participate in contact sports or high-velocity ball sports. These injuries require early and appropriate treatment to avoid stiffness and long-term dysfunction. Although closed reduction and immobilization are appropriate for some injuries, early reduction and fixation in some cases allows for less time out of sport, and should be considered in select circumstances.

Condylar fractures
Not uncommonly, athletes sustain injuries to their hands resulting in fractured condyles. Unicondylar fractures can occur when balls strike separated, outstretched digits at high velocity.[27,28] These injuries are very unstable, and require close follow-up, often requiring internal fixation.[28] With stable fixation, athletes can initiate early motion and return to competition within 1 week, with buddy-tape protection.[27]

Shaft fractures
Although minimally displaced phalangeal shaft fractures can often be treated safely with buddy taping and early mobilization, some phalangeal shaft fractures may best be treated with surgical stabilization. Owing to the deforming forces across the phalanx, fractures may have significant angulation. In the proximal phalanx, shaft fractures tend to present with apex–volar angulation, owing to the flexion force of the intrinsics on the proximal fragment, and the extension force of the extensor mechanism across the distal fragment.

Plate fixation may be recommended for some patients presenting with phalangeal shaft fractures, when they present with comminution, multiple fractures, or significant transverse displacement.[27] Although tendon glide is a concern with placement of hardware on the phalanges, a midaxial approach and low-profile plate helps to minimize this problem.[27] For long oblique or spiral fractures of the phalanx, lag screws can hold a fracture in a reduced position, while again causing minimal trauma to the nearby tendons.[27] Both techniques allow early motion and minimize time away from sport.

Distal Phalanx Fractures

Distal phalanx fractures can be the result of a direct blow or, more commonly, a crushing mechanism. When these fractures occur, they can occur with or without an injury to the nail bed. Often, when nail bed injuries occur with distal phalanx fractures, these require nail plate removal, irrigation, and nail bed repair to limit the chances of infection. However, most simple distal phalanx fractures can be treated with simple splinting in a protected position, with early return to sport. Fingertip protectors may allow athletes to return comfortably to sport. In certain cases, distal phalanx fractures may be associated with tendon injuries, known as mallet finger or jersey finger. These conditions, which are discussed in detail elsewhere in this article, should be recognized and treated appropriately.

Proximal Interphalangeal Joint Dislocations

Dorsal proximal interphalangeal joint dislocations are the most common hand injury among athletes.[29] Many proximal interphalangeal dislocations can be treated with early reduction and buddy taping to an adjacent finger for 3 to 6 weeks with early motion. Return to play may be allowed during this time as pain and swelling permit.[4] Some proximal interphalangeal dislocations are associated with fractures of the base of P2. These injuries should be carefully evaluated for instability or persistent subluxation. If unable to be corrected to a well-aligned joint, these may require formal open reduction and internal fixation.[29] For missed injuries or acute injuries that are not amenable to primary repair, techniques such as the hemihamate autograft have been used successfully (**Fig. 4**).[30] Unstable injuries should be treated with cessation of sports for 4 weeks.[4]

THUMB ULNAR COLLATERAL LIGAMENT INJURY

Injuries to the thumb ulnar collateral ligament (UCL) can occur in any sport, with abduction and forced radial deviation. It is classically known as "skier's thumb" because it is associated with injury to the ligament as the thumb is stressed against a ski pole.[4] Patients present with swelling and bruising about the base of the thumb, and gapping or laxity of the joint on stress examination (**Fig. 5**).

Stable injuries to the UCL, which present as nondisplaced avulsion fractures, may be treated nonoperatively in a cast. Unstable injuries, however, require operative intervention to repair or reconstruct the UCL. This is typically done through a dorsal/ulnar approach, after which the adductor aponeurosis is taken down to allow visualization of the UCL (**Fig. 6**). The UCL is typically avulsed off of the base of the metacarpal, and can be repaired back to this surface using suture anchors. After either

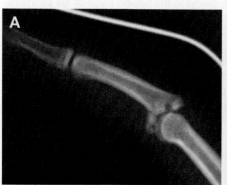
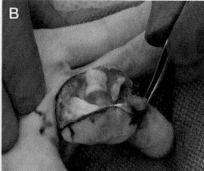
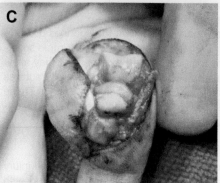

Fig. 4. A professional football player sustained an injury to his proximal interphalangeal joint. (*A*) Proximal interphalangeal fracture–dislocation. (*B, C*) Intraoperative photographs demonstrate the bone loss at the base of the second phalanx. Bone loss and articular contour are repaired using a hemihamate autograft.

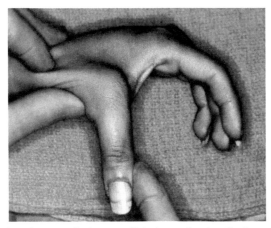

Fig. 5. Intraoperative photograph shows a clinical examination finding confirming rupture of the thumb ulnar collateral ligament.

intervention, athletes can return to sport immediately with appropriate immobilization. Noncontact athletes must wear thumb spica casts or thermoplastic splints for 4 weeks, whereas athletes involved in contact sports should be casted for 4 weeks with an additional 2 weeks of splinting.[4]

JERSEY FINGER AND MALLET FINGER
Jersey Finger

An avulsion of the flexor digitorum profundus from the insertion point on the distal phalanx is known as jersey finger. It gets its name from the classic mechanism, of a forced extension on a flexed as a player grabs another player's jersey.[31] It is observed most commonly in the ring finger, but can occur in any digit. The injury can be associated with a bony fragment or can be purely ligamentous.

Repair of these injuries is nearly universally indicated, because nonoperative management typically results in permanent disability or necessitates later fusion of the distal interphalangeal joint. The flexor digitorum profundus tendon may retract as far proximally as the palm, which indicates disruption of blood supply and increases the urgency of repair. In general, tendons should be repaired as early as possible to minimize scar adhesion and contraction.

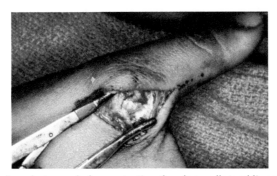

Fig. 6. Intraoperative photograph demonstrating the ulnar collateral ligament avulsed from the first metacarpal.

Postoperatively, active flexion is limited and occupational therapy are necessary to promote tendon excursion, minimize scar tissue, and protect the repair.[31] Return to play for contact sports or ball or racket sports may not be appropriate before 4 to 6 months postoperatively.[31]

Mallet Finger

Avulsions of the extensor tendon from its origin on the distal phalanx are known as mallet finger. Patients present after forced flexion or axial load against a hyperextended finger, with the distal interphalangeal joint positioned in flexion with inability to actively extend. These injuries, unlike jersey finger, are often successfully treated nonoperatively. A variety of immobilization techniques have been designed (see **Fig. 6**):

- Stack splint
- QuickCast
- Alumifoam splinting (dorsal or volar)
- Custom thermoplastic splints

None of these immobilization techniques has been shown to be significantly advantageous over the other.[32] However, patient compliance with brace wear is crucial to the success of immobilization.[33]

Return to play may be initiated immediately when splinting begins, depending on pain and requirements of the sport. Typically, at least 6 weeks of immobilization is necessary. Although some practitioners advocate additional nighttime splinting after 6 weeks, no definitive data support the need for this measure.

SUMMARY/DISCUSSION

Hand and wrist injuries affect a huge number of athletes each year. It is important to initiate early and appropriate treatment for each injury, and to find a reasonable balance between allowing bony and soft tissue healing and encouraging early range of motion and return to activity. In many cases, athletes may return to sport with protective immobilization and close follow-up. It is up to the physician to determine which patients are appropriate for early return to play, based on their athletic participation and the nature of their injury. Professional athletes and those who depend heavily on their sporting ability should generally be returned to sport as soon as safely allowed. Playing casts and immobilization may allow early return, and should be considered strongly when the athlete's livelihood and career are at stake. Collegiate athletes should be returned to sport similarly aggressively, depending on their division and investment in their sport. However, high school and recreational athletes should generally be treated more cautiously, because reinjury in this population will be less well-tolerated by patients and their parents, given that early return to sport is not as crucial and does not merit the risk of reinjury. The treating physician must carefully weigh all of these factors. Counseling in many cases may be among the most important aspects of the patient visit, especially balancing expectations for return to sport and disability. Ideally, patients return to sport in a safe and reasonable timeframe, understanding the likelihood of reinjury and full recovery.

REFERENCES

1. Rettig AC, Patel DV. Epidemiology of elbow, forearm, and wrist injuries in the athlete. Clin Sports Med 1995;14(2):289–97.
2. Rettig AC. Epidemiology of hand and wrist injuries in sports. Clin Sports Med 1998;17(3):401–6.

3. Lawson GM, Hajducka C, McQueen MM. Sports fractures of the distal radius–epidemiology and outcome. Injury 1995;26(1):33–6.
4. Morgan WJ, Slowman LS. Acute hand and wrist injuries in athletes: evaluation and management. J Am Acad Orthop Surg 2001;9(6):389–400.
5. Eddeland A, Eiken O, Hellgren E, et al. Fractures of the scaphoid. Scand J Plast Reconstr Surg 1975;9(3):234–9.
6. Jorgensen TM, Andresen JH, Thommesen P, et al. Scanning and radiology of the carpal scaphoid bone. Acta Orthop Scand 1979;50(6 Pt 1):663–5.
7. Kukla C, Gaebler C, Breitenseher MJ, et al. Occult fractures of the scaphoid. The diagnostic usefulness and indirect economic repercussions of radiography versus magnetic resonance scanning. J Hand Surg Br 1997;22(6):810–3.
8. Kumar S, O'Connor A, Despois M, et al. Use of early magnetic resonance imaging in the diagnosis of occult scaphoid fractures: the CAST Study (Canberra Area Scaphoid Trial). N Z Med J 2005;118(1209):U1296.
9. Patel NK, Davies N, Mirza Z, et al. Cost and clinical effectiveness of MRI in occult scaphoid fractures: a randomised controlled trial. Emerg Med J 2013;30(3):202–7.
10. Clay NR, Dias JJ, Costigan PS, et al. Need the thumb be immobilised in scaphoid fractures? A randomised prospective trial. J Bone Joint Surg Br 1991;73(5):828–32.
11. Rettig AC, Weidenbener EJ, Gloyeske R. Alternative management of midthird scaphoid fractures in the athlete. Am J Sports Med 1994;22(5):711–4.
12. Riester JN, Baker BE, Mosher JF, et al. A review of scaphoid fracture healing in competitive athletes. Am J Sports Med 1985;13(3):159–61.
13. Bond CD, Shin AY, McBride MT, et al. Percutaneous screw fixation or cast immobilization for nondisplaced scaphoid fractures. J Bone Joint Surg Am 2001;83A(4):483–8.
14. Slade JF 3rd, Milewski MD. Management of carpal instability in athletes. Hand Clin 2009;25(3):395–408.
15. Devers BN, Douglas KC, Naik RD, et al. Outcomes of hook of hamate fracture excision in high-level amateur athletes. J Hand Surg Am 2013;38(1):72–6.
16. Parker RD, Berkowitz MS, Brahms MA, et al. Hook of the hamate fractures in athletes. Am J Sports Med 1986;14(6):517–23.
17. Lewis DM, Osterman AL. Scapholunate instability in athletes. Clin Sports Med 2001;20(1):131–40, ix.
18. Lavernia CJ, Cohen MS, Taleisnik J. Treatment of scapholunate dissociation by ligamentous repair and capsulodesis. J Hand Surg Am 1992;17(2):354–9.
19. Williams A, Ng CY, Hayton MJ. When can a professional athlete return to play following scapholunate ligament delayed reconstruction? Br J Sports Med 2013;47(17):1071–4.
20. Tavassoli J, Ruland RT, Hogan CJ, et al. Three cast techniques for the treatment of extra-articular metacarpal fractures. Comparison of short-term outcomes and final fracture alignments. J Bone Joint Surg Am 2005;87(10):2196–201.
21. Toronto R, Donovan PJ, Macintyre J. An alternative method of treatment for metacarpal fractures in athletes. Clin J Sport Med 1996;6(1):4–8.
22. van Aaken J, Kampfen S, Berli M, et al. Outcome of boxer's fractures treated by a soft wrap and buddy taping: a prospective study. Hand (N Y) 2007;2(4):212–7.
23. Statius Muller MG, Poolman RW, van Hoogstraten MJ, et al. Immediate mobilization gives good results in boxer's fractures with volar angulation up to 70 degrees: a prospective randomized trial comparing immediate mobilization with cast immobilization. Arch Orthop Trauma Surg 2003;123(10):534–7.

24. Fisher MR, Rogers LF, Hendrix RW. Systematic approach to identifying fourth and fifth carpometacarpal joint dislocations. AJR Am J Roentgenol 1983;140(2): 319–24.
25. Zhang C, Wang H, Liang C, et al. The effect of timing on the treatment and outcome of combined fourth and fifth carpometacarpal fracture dislocations. J Hand Surg Am 2015;40(11):2169–75.e1.
26. Lawlis JF 3rd, Gunther SF. Carpometacarpal dislocations. Long-term follow-up. J Bone Joint Surg Am 1991;73(1):52–9.
27. Geissler WB. Operative fixation of metacarpal and phalangeal fractures in athletes. Hand Clin 2009;25(3):409–21.
28. Weiss AP, Hastings H 2nd. Distal unicondylar fractures of the proximal phalanx. J Hand Surg Am 1993;18(4):594–9.
29. Palmer RE. Joint injuries of the hand in athletes. Clin Sports Med 1998;17(3): 513–31.
30. Williams RM, Kiefhaber TR, Sommerkamp TG, et al. Treatment of unstable dorsal proximal interphalangeal fracture/dislocations using a hemi-hamate autograft. J Hand Surg Am 2003;28(5):856–65.
31. Kovacic J, Bergfeld J. Return to play issues in upper extremity injuries. Clin J Sport Med 2005;15(6):448–52.
32. Valdes K, Naughton N, Algar L. Conservative treatment of mallet finger: a systematic review. J Hand Ther 2015;28(3):237–45 [quiz: 246].
33. Groth GN, Wilder DM, Young VL. The impact of compliance on the rehabilitation of patients with mallet finger injuries. J Hand Ther 1994;7(1):21–4.

Return to Play After Lumbar Spine Surgery

Ralph W. Cook, BS[1], Wellington K. Hsu, MD*

KEYWORDS

- Athlete • Return to play • Lumbar spine injury • Lumbar spine surgery
- Performance outcomes

KEY POINTS

- Surgical management of selected lumbar spine conditions can produce excellent outcomes in athletes of all sports.
- Microdiscectomy for lumbar disc herniation has been the most well-studied procedure and leads to favorable outcomes in return to play rates and statistical performance postoperatively.
- Direct pars repair has led to high rates of return to play for a variety of fixation techniques.
- There is a paucity of evidence-based return to play criteria, with the majority of literature based on expert opinion and clinical experience.

INTRODUCTION

Low back pain (LBP) is one of the most common chief complaints encountered in medicine, affecting 80% of the general population at some point in life. Athletes are also commonly afflicted, with incidence rates approaching 30% over the course of a career, accounting for one of the most common reasons for missed playing time.[1,2] In fact, 38% of professional tennis players reported missing at least 1 tournament owing to LBP at some point during their career.[3] A survey of 272 competitive adolescent athletes involved in 31 different sports found a point prevalence (within the last 48 hours) of LBP of 14%, a 1-year prevalence of 57%, and a lifetime

Disclosures: Consulting - Stryker, Bacterin, Graftys, Globus, AONA, Synthes, Spinesmith, SI Bone, Relievant, Ceramtec, Medtronic, Pioneer, Bioventus, LifeNet. Speaking and/or Teaching Arrangements - AONA. Trips/travel - Stryker, Pioneer Surgical, Medtronic, Bioventus, AONA. Board of Directors - Lumbar Spine Research Society, Cervical Spine Research Society. Scientific Advisory Board - Bioventus (W.K. Hsu); none (R.W. Cook).
Source of Funding: There was no external source of funding for this project.
Department of Orthopaedic Surgery, Northwestern University Feinberg School of Medicine, Northwestern University, 676 North Saint Clair Street, Suite 1350, Chicago, IL 60611, USA
[1] Present address: 6 Buck Run, Mohnton, PA 19540.
* Corresponding author.
E-mail address: wkhsu@yahoo.com

prevalence of 66%.[4] Additionally, a study examining the medical records of 4790 inter-collegiate athletes competing in 17 varsity sports over a 10-year period revealed a spine injury rate of 7 per 100 participants.[5]

Spine problems can be associated with participation in sports involving repetitive hyperextension, flexion, rotation, and axial loading, such as gymnastics, wrestling, football, diving, soccer, and dance.[2,5-7] Overuse injuries have been found to be more common than acute ones in a young athletic population.[6] Furthermore, the diagnoses given to athletes differ depending on an athlete's age. One study compared adolescent athletes with adults with acute LBP and demonstrated that 47% of adolescents had stress fractures of the pars interarticularis, compared with only 5% of adults.[8] Conversely, discogenic back pain was diagnosed in 48% of adults compared with only 11% of adolescents.

Initial treatment for a lumbar spine injury consists of conservative management, including a brief period of rest and cessation of sporting activity for 1 to 2 days.[9] Medications may consist of nonsteroidal antiinflammatory drugs and muscle relaxants. Physical therapy modalities such as ice, heat, compression, and massage may bring additional pain relief. Certain injuries, such as lumbar disc herniation, may benefit from lumbar epidural corticosteroid injections. Once pain has been controlled successfully, activity may be resumed after a short course of flexibility and strengthening exercises. Return to play, in general, should be considered when an athlete is pain free, has full active range of motion with all activities, and has normal strength, endurance, and flexibility.[2,6,9,10] Although conservative management can often lead to pain relief in the majority of patients, those who fail this treatment may require surgery.

Outcome measures used to judge success in the general population may not be specific enough for professional athletes, who must return to play at a high level for their livelihood. Validated patient reported outcome measures such as visual analog scales, the Oswestry Disability Index, and the Short Form-36 may not be as applicable to athletes, who are interested in returning to their preinjury level of performance and on career longevity. More recently, clinical studies have focused on return to play and sport-specific performance based outcome measures after treatment for lumbar spine injury. Nonetheless, there is substantial variability in published return to play criteria, which are almost exclusively derived from author's expert opinion and experience.[9,11] This article summarizes the current literature that defines return to play criteria for various lumbar spine injuries.

LUMBAR DISC HERNIATION

For athletes who fail conservative management, lumbar discectomy provides symptom relief and improved functional outcomes in the vast majority of patients.[12] For example, in 14 division I athletes in the National Collegiate Athletic Association from 1988 to 1995, 90% of all athletes undergoing single level microdiscectomy returned to varsity sports, with all athletes returning to at least recreational sporting activities.[13] Recently, a systematic review that included 10 studies found that 75% to 100% of elite athletes return to play after operative treatment for lumbar disc herniation.[14] The recovery period after surgery ranged from 2.8 to 8.7 months, with athletes' postoperative careers ranging from 2.6 to 4.8 years. Notably, elite athletes attained an average of 64% to 104% of preoperative baseline statistics, with variable performance based on sport. Similarly, a metaanalysis performed by Overley and colleagues[15] evaluated 9 studies representing 558 patients with lumbar disc herniation who underwent lumbar microdiscectomy. The pooled clinical success rate (defined as logging playing time in at least 1 regular season game or Olympic-level event) for return to play after operative treatment was 83.5%.

In a multidisciplinary effort from Northwestern University called the Professional Athlete Spine Initiative, outcomes after lumbar disc herniation in 342 professional athletes from the 4 major North American sports (baseball, basketball, American football, and hockey) from 1972 to 2008 were studied.[16] Successful return to play, defined as return to the active roster for at least 1 professional regular season game after treatment, was found to be 82%, with an average career length of 3.4 years after lumbar disc herniation. There was no difference between operative and nonoperative cohorts (81% return to play for 3.3 years and 84% for 3.5 years, respectively). Older age at diagnosis was a negative predictor of career duration after injury, whereas a greater number of professional games played before injury had positive effects on outcomes. Furthermore, there was significant variability in return to play rates between sports, with Major League Baseball players having a significantly higher return to play rate compared with other sports, and National Football League (NFL) athletes have significantly lower return to play rates. Subgroup analysis demonstrated that NFL athletes had the greatest treatment effect from surgery, whereas microdiscectomy in Major League Baseball players led to significantly shorter careers compared with nonoperative controls. The authors concluded that the differing inherent physical demands of particular sports may affect return to play rates for athletes.

American Football

Although the physical demands from a collision sport such as American football should be considered when treating athletes of this sport, in a study of 137 NFL players from 1978 to 2008, Hsu[17] demonstrated the potential beneficial effect of surgery for lumbar disc herniation compared with conservative management. Return to play rates were not different between operative and nonoperative groups (78% vs 59%, respectively); however, players treated operatively played in significantly more games postoperatively (n = 36) than those treated nonoperatively (n = 20). There were potential confounding variables; the nonoperative group was significantly older than the operative cohort. Subsequently, a subgroup analysis evaluated outcomes in offensive and defensive linemen—players generally considered to be at the greatest risk for lumbar disc herniation.[18] In this group of players that are constantly subjected to bodily impact in a crouched/stooped position on every play, 81% of surgically treated players return to play an average of 33 games over 3.0 years compared with only 29% of nonoperative players for 5.1 games over 0.8 years. In operatively treated players, 14% of linemen required a revision microdiscectomy, with 6 of 7 athletes returning to play afterward, suggesting that this procedure is not a contraindication for return to play in this population. In another subgroup analysis of offensive skill position players (quarterback, running back, wide receiver, and tight end), 74% of athletes return to play for an average of 36 games over 4.1 years, with no statistically significant difference in performance between preinjury and postinjury statistics.[19] These studies suggest that surgical management for lumbar disc herniation in NFL athletes have generally favorable return to play rates, with little impact on performance.

Baseball

The constant requirements of twisting and axial rotation of baseball athletes during hitting and pitching may lead to different outcomes after lumbar surgery in this patient population. In a biomechanical analysis of elite baseball players, the greatest amount of force generated during batting occurred after ball contact and during pitching near front foot contact.[20] The authors suggested that these forces may lead to greater intradiscal pressures, which may predispose these athletes to either virgin or recurrent lumbar spine injuries. In a study of 69 lumbar disc herniation in 64 Major League

Baseball athletes, 97% successfully return to play at an average of 6.6 months after diagnosis.[21] Athletes treated operatively required significantly more time to return to play than those managed conservatively (8.7 vs 3.6 months, respectively).[21] In contrast with studies in other sports,[19,22] pitchers and hitters demonstrated significantly poorer performance in certain vital statistical categories postoperatively, whereas the nonoperative cohort returned to play at preoperative performance levels and with longer careers.[16,21]

Basketball

Anakwenze and colleagues[12] evaluated 24 NBA athletes who underwent lumbar discectomy for lumbar disc herniation between 1991 and 2007. After surgery, 75% successfully return to play, with a significant increase in blocked shots per 40 minutes and a smaller decrease in rebounds per 40 minutes when compared with age and position matched controls at 1 year after surgery. More recently, Minhas and colleagues[22] evaluated 61 NBA players with lumbar disc herniation, demonstrating that return to play rates did not differ between operatively and nonoperatively treated players (78% vs 79%, respectively). Using a novel method for historical, comparable players as controls, athletes' careers with lumbar disc herniation were compared with similar ones without this diagnosis. During the first postindex season, operatively treated athletes played in significantly fewer games and had lower player efficiency ratings compared with controls; however, no difference was seen at 2 and 3 years after surgery or in postoperative career length. Conversely, whereas athletes managed conservatively showed no difference at any time point in games played or player efficiency ratings compared with controls, they did tend to play significantly fewer postindex seasons.

Hockey

Schroeder and colleagues[23] investigated 87 National Hockey League players with lumbar disc herniation, of which 31 underwent nonoperative treatment, 48 received a discectomy, and 8 were treated with a single level fusion. Return to play for all players was 85% for an average of 136 games over 2.7 years. There was no difference in return to play rates between those treated surgically (82%) and conservatively (90%); however, all players had a significant decrease in performance measures after lumbar disc herniation (games per season, points per game, and performance score) with no difference between treatment groups. The lumbar fusion group returned to play 100% of the time for an average of 203 games over 4 years, with no decrease in performance measures. The authors warned that this difference could be attributed to the small sample size of the fusion cohort; however, this limited evidence suggests that lumbar fusion may be compatible with return to play in the National Hockey League, which remains a relative contraindication in other collision sports. Overall, this study intimates that National Hockey League athletes with lumbar disc herniation can expect some decline in performance after injury.

These studies suggest excellent return to play rates and variable posttreatment performance depending on the sport played; however, time to return is not always clear and differences in methodology make comparing results difficult. Watkins and colleagues[24] initially evaluated 60 cases of microdiscectomy in 59 Olympic and professional athletes with lumbar disc herniation between 1984 and 1998. They found that 90% return to play at an average of 5.2 months (range, 1–15). Watkins and associates[25] later attempted to better define the timeline for return in 171 professional athletes between 1996 to 2010 based on in-season eligibility criteria. They found that, overall, 89% of surgically treated patients return to play at an average of 5.8 months.

Furthermore, 50% returned at 3 months, increasing to 72% at 6 months, 77% at 9 months, and 84% at 12 months.

There is a paucity of evidence-based return to play criteria after surgery for lumbar disc herniation in the literature, with all of the recommendations published to date based exclusively on authors' expert opinion (**Table 1**). Generally speaking, patients must be symptom free, have full active range of motion, and be near full strength before returning to sports activities.[2,6,9] There are no contraindications after lumbar discectomy for return to any sport.[11,26–28]

SPONDYLOLYSIS AND SPONDYLOLISTHESIS

Spondylolysis and spondylolisthesis are among the most common causes of LBP in adolescents, with rates as high as 47% reported in the literature.[8] Participation in sports involving repetitive hyperextension, rotation, axial loading, and torsion against resistance predispose young athletes to stress fractures of the pars interarticularis.[2,7,29] Radiographic analysis of 100 young female gymnasts (average age 14 years) engaged in high-level competition revealed a prevalence of spondylolysis in 11%.[30] Furthermore, prevalence rates are particularly high among athletes engaged in diving (43%), wrestling (30%), throwing sports (27%), weight lifting (23%), artistic gymnastics (17%), and rowing (17%).[29,31]

Nonoperative treatment for acute spondylolysis, consisting of activity restriction and bracing for up to 6 months, results in successful pain relief in more than 80% of athletes independent of radiographic evidence of defect healing.[2] When conservative measures fail, direct surgical repair or posterolateral fusion can yield high rates of pain relief and enable return to play. Direct pars repair may be more advantageous for athletes and facilitate higher return to play rates, because it preserves spinal motion.[9] Several techniques exist, including the Buck screw, Scott wiring technique, and Morscher hook screw.

A systematic review encompassing 84 young amateur athletes (mean age 20 years) found that most pars fractures occurred at the L5 vertebral level (96%), and that 84% of operatively treated athletes return to play at their preinjury level of intensity over the course of 5 to 12 months after direct pars repair.[7] Of the 13 who were unable to return to play, 7 were able to return to a less strenuous sport. A more recent comprehensive review reporting on the surgical and conservative treatment of spondylolysis and low-grade spondylolisthesis in competitive amateur athletes from 1973 to 2014 found return to play rates of 88% and 85% for surgical and conservative treatment, respectively, over 6 to 12 months.[32] Of note, direct pars repair led to 80% to 100% return to play rates in the studies analyzed, representing an excellent treatment option for young athletes.

Table 1
Recommendations for RTP after discectomy and microdiscectomy

Treatment	Type of Sport	RTP Recommendation	Author, Year
Percutaneous discectomy	All sports	2–3 mo[28]	Eck & Riley,[28] 2004
Microdiscectomy (adult)	Golf	4–8 wk[41]	Abla et al,[41] 2011
	Noncontact sports	6–8 wk[28]	Eck & Riley,[28] 2004
	Contact sports	4–6 mo[28]	Eck & Riley,[28] 2004
	Contact sports	2–6 mo[11]	Huang et al,[11] 2016
Microdiscectomy (pediatric)	All sports	8–12 wk[27]	Cahill et al,[27] 2010

Abbreviation: RTP, return to play.

With the Buck screw technique in 25 competitive athletes, there was a 76% return to play rate at a mean of 6 months (range, 3–10) after surgery.[33] Similarly, of 16 adolescent patients with 29 pars defects treated using Buck screw placement, 94% had symptom resolution, with a 97% overall fusion rate.[34] Of the 8 athletes in this cohort, 100% successfully returned to play. Finally, Debnath and colleagues[35] evaluated 19 young athletes who underwent operative treatment for lumbar spondylolysis with Buck screw fixation, reporting 95% return to play at a mean of 7 months (range, 4–10).

Using a Scott wire fixation technique, Nozawa and colleagues[36] reported outcomes in 20 athletes after surgery for spondylolysis. All of these athletes were able to return to play, although to varying degrees after surgery, demonstrating that excellent results can be obtained with this method of fixation. In 1 study of 43 adolescent athletes treated with the Morscher hook screw construct for spondylolysis or grade I spondylolisthesis, 100% were able to return to play after 4 months after surgery.[37] Similarly, in a study of 5 intercollegiate athletes with acute lumbar spondylolysis undergoing direct pars repair with the hook screw construct, 100% return to play within 6 months after diagnosis.[38] A recent trend using novel, minimally invasive techniques to treat pars fractures has become more prevalent.[39] One such method involves placement of pedicle screws connected to a radiolucent cord placed under tension through 2 bilateral stab incisions 3 cm paramedian to the midline. In 1 study using this technique, 8 athletes of varying levels of competition with 16 pars defects underwent minimally invasive surgery to repair the defect. Of these, 75% returned to play at their previous level of competition after 6 months, and all patients reported overall mean improvements in validated patient-reported outcome measures.

Evidence-based return to play criteria are also limited in the present literature for spondylolysis and spondylolisthesis, with all available guidelines based exclusively on expert opinion (**Tables 2** and **3**). Although authors may disagree on the timing and possibility of return for certain sports, there is a general consensus that those who return to play should be pain free with nearly normal strength, flexibility, and endurance.[2,10,26] Furthermore, those who undergo lumbar fusion should have radiographic evidence of solid bony fusion; however, this is not necessarily as critical for those requiring direct pars repair.[2,10,26,36]

There is also general agreement that before return to play, athletes should complete a postoperative physical therapy and rehabilitation program.[9] Radcliff and colleagues[10] described a rehabilitation protocol for patients recovering from direct pars repair. In it, they recommend a program of supervised core strengthening, flexibility work for the extremities, and water exercises performed with a neutral spine beginning at 2 weeks postoperatively. Nonimpact aerobic activities may commence 2 to 4 weeks postoperatively, with a neutral spine for up to the first 3 months. Gradual impact and dynamic exercises were added at 3 months, with sport-specific training

Table 2		
Recommendations for RTP after direct pars repair		
Type of Sport	**RTP Recommendation**	**Author, Year**
Contact sports	Allowed, but no defined timeframe[36]	Nozawa et al,[36] 2003
Contact sports	6 mo[39]	Gillis et al,[39] 2015
Contact sports	6–12 mo[10]	Radcliff et al,[10] 2009
Contact sports	6–12 mo[32]	Bouras & Korovessis,[32] 2015
Collision sports	Allowed, but no defined timeframe[36]	Nozawa et al,[36] 2003

Abbreviation: RTP, return to play.

Table 3
Recommendations for RTP after lumbar fusion

Type of Sport	RTP Recommendation	Author, Year
Golf	6 mo[41]	Abla et al,[41] 2011
Noncontact sports	6–12 mo[40]	Rubery & Bradford,[40] 2002
Noncontact sports	12 mo[28]	Eck & Riley,[28] 2004
Noncontact sports (scoliosis)	4 mo[44]	Fabricant et al,[44] 2012
Contact sports	12 mo[40]	Rubery & Bradford,[40] 2002
Contact sports	6–12 mo[32]	Bouras & Korovessis,[32] 2015
Contact sports	Not recommended[28]	Eck & Riley,[28] 2004
Collision sports	Not recommended[32]	Bouras & Korovessis,[32] 2015
Collision sports	Not recommended[11]	Huang et al,[11] 2016

Abbreviation: RTP, return to play.

following at 4 to 6 months. The ultimate goal of this protocol is for return to play to contact sports at 6 to 12 months after surgery. Similarly, Gillis and colleagues[39] recommended return to high impact activities at 6 months, and Nozawa and colleagues[36] recommend that patients should be allowed to return to contact and collision sports after surgery if they show evidence of rigid bony union on plain radiographic films or computed tomography scan.

For posterolateral fusion for spondylolysis/spondylolisthesis, there are many surgeons who would allow eventual return to noncontact but not collision sports.[40] Conversely, others have supported their patients return to contact sports after lumbar fusion.[26,28,32,40,41] Rubery and Bradford[40] conducted a poll of 261 Scoliosis Research Society members to determine return to play recommendation patterns for different lumbar spine pathologies. The data suggested that a majority of surgeons would recommend returning to contact sports at 1 year after lumbar fusion for both low- and high-grade spondylolisthesis (56% and 51%, respectively). Interestingly, 12% to 15% of respondents would advise against and 2% to 6% would forbid return to contact sports in this population. In a separate study, Bouras and Korovessis[32] allowed return to contact sports after lumbar fusion for spondylolisthesis within 1 year of surgery; however, they strictly forbade return to sports such as gymnastics, football, rugby, wrestling, weight lifting, skydiving, and bungee jumping. In contrast, Eck and Riley[28] were more conservative, recommending against return to contact sports.

DEGENERATIVE DISC DISEASE

Degenerative disc disease (DDD) is a common finding in athletes with LBP.[2] Older athletes are at an increased risk of developing back pain secondary to DDD with 48% of patients given this diagnosis in one study.[8] Although conservative management is always the first line of treatment for this patient population, it is possible that chronic pain recalcitrant to nonoperative modalities may be treated successfully with surgery in selected athletes.[2]

Although there are no studies that evaluate lumbar fusion for DDD in an athletic population, recent literature has looked at outcomes of total disc replacement (TDR) in the active competitive athlete and military population.[42,43] One study evaluated 39 athletes (average age 39.8 years) treated with TDR for DDD.[42] These athletes return to play 95% of the time to all sports, with subjective full recovery and peak fitness noted after 5.2 months. The authors returned their patients to all contact and/or extreme sports without restrictions. In 8% of patients, persistent LBP limited physical activity.

Another study compared TDR with anterior lumbar interbody fusion in 24 active duty military personnel (average age 37.3 years).[43] TDR patients returned to full active duty 83% (10/12) of the time, at an average of 22.6 weeks, whereas anterior lumbar interbody fusion patients returned 67% (8/12) of the time at an average of 32.4 weeks postoperatively ($P = .156$). The authors note that return-to-action criteria may have been affected by confounding factors, such as radiographic criteria after fusion. These studies suggest that TDR may be a viable alternative to lumbar fusion for the treatment of DDD in this population.

At best, there is level V evidence to guide return to play recommendations after surgical treatment for lumbar DDD (see **Table 3**; **Tables 4** and **5**). Many authors suggest that, before considering return to play, an athlete should have radiographic evidence of a solid fusion, resolution of preoperative pain, and restoration of strength, flexibility, and endurance.[2] A survey of North American Spine Society members revealed that a majority of respondents would recommend a return to golf no sooner than 6 months after lumbar spine fusion.[41] Although many respondents allowed significantly shorter recovery times for professional compared with noncompetitive golfers, they stressed the importance of fusion healing and evidence of radiographic stability. Siepe and colleagues[42] recommended athlete participation in noncontact sports within 3 months of TDR, and that contact and even extreme sports may be resumed after 4 to 6 months. Tumialan and colleagues[43] support nonimpact training starting at 3 months, with no activity limitations after 6 months after TDR surgery. After a laminectomy alone for spinal stenosis, Abla and colleagues[41] suggest that athletes may resume golf after 4 to 8 weeks, whereas 2 other studies suggest that participation in contact sports may commence 4 to 6 months postoperatively.[11,28]

ADOLESCENT IDIOPATHIC SCOLIOSIS

Adolescent idiopathic scoliosis can cause LBP in the athletic population, and in certain situations, surgery is indicated to halt the progression of the curvature. One study to date has evaluated return to play outcomes in 42 athletically active adolescents with scoliosis who underwent posterior spinal fusion.[44] The authors report that 60% of children returned to play contact and noncontact sports at an equal or higher level of activity postoperatively. There was a significant relationship between the distal level of fusion and the rate of return to play—the lower the level of instrumentation from T11 to L4, the lower the return to play rate, with calculated odds ratios indicating that for each level fused distally, patients were 36.7% less likely to return to play at or above the same level of preoperative activity ($P = .039$). Furthermore, higher Lenke

---

Table 4
Recommendations for RTP after laminectomy

Type of Sport	RTP Recommendation	Author, Year
Golf	4–8 wk[41]	Abla et al,[41] 2011
Contact sports	4–6 mo[28]	Eck & Riley,[28] 2004
Contact sports	4–6 mo[11]	Huang et al,[11] 2016
Contact sports	Allowed, but no defined time frame[26]	Burnett & Sonntag,[26] 2006
Collision sports	Not recommended[11]	Huang et al,[11] 2016

Abbreviation: RTP, return to play.

Table 5
Recommendations for RTP after lumbar total disc replacement

Type of Sport	RTP Recommendation	Author, Year
Noncontact sports	3 mo[42]	Siepe et al,[42] 2007
Nonimpact training	3 mo[43]	Tumialan et al,[43] 2010
Light impact training	4–5 mo[43]	Tumialan et al,[43] 2010
Unrestricted duty	6 mo[43]	Tumialan et al,[43] 2010
Contact sports	4–6 mo[42]	Siepe et al,[42] 2007

Abbreviation: RTP, return to play.

classification curve types and lower final Scoliosis Research Society-22 scores were also negative predictors of return to play rates. The data in this study suggests that fusion for adolescent idiopathic scoliosis may have negative consequences on return to play for young athletes, which also depends on the extent of the surgery.

As far as time to return to play is concerned, some have recommended return to play at 4 months after surgery if patients were pain free with radiographic evidence that the implants and curve correction remained unchanged[44] (see **Table 3**). In this particular study, clearance was granted at an average of 7.4 months postoperatively. A Scoliosis Research Society survey study reported that a majority of respondents supported return to noncontact sports at 6 months after fusion for adolescent idiopathic scoliosis, with 61% of respondents supporting return to contact sports at 1 year.[40] Interestingly, collision sports were allowed by 32% of respondents, with the vast majority advising against (36%) or forbidding (24%) them.

SUMMARY

Surgical management of lumbar spine conditions can produce excellent outcomes in athletes. Microdiscectomy for lumbar disc herniation has exceptionally favorable outcomes, with the vast majority of athletes returning to play a wide variety of sports with little impact on performance measures. Direct pars repair is equally successful in younger athletes, with high rates of return to play for a variety of fixation techniques. There is a paucity of evidence based return to play criteria, with the majority of literature based on expert opinion and clinical experience. Athletes should demonstrate full resolution of symptoms, along with adequate flexibility, endurance, and strength before return to play. Physicians' decisions on when to return an athlete to sport should be dependent on the particular injury sustained, chosen sport, and individual factors.

REFERENCES

1. Dreisinger TE, Nelson B. Management of back pain in athletes. Sports Med 1996; 21(4):313–20.
2. Bono CM. Low-back pain in athletes. J Bone Joint Surg Am 2004;86A(2):382–96.
3. Hainline B. Low back injury. Clin Sports Med 1995;14(1):241–65.
4. Schmidt CP, Zwingenberger S, Walther A, et al. Prevalence of low back pain in adolescent athletes - an epidemiological investigation. Int J Sports Med 2014; 35(8):684–9.
5. Keene JS, Albert MJ, Springer SL, et al. Back injuries in college athletes. J Spinal Disord 1989;2(3):190–5.
6. Purcell L, Micheli L. Low back pain in young athletes. Sports Health 2009;1(3): 212–22.

7. Drazin D, Shirzadi A, Jeswani S, et al. Direct surgical repair of spondylolysis in athletes: indications, techniques, and outcomes. Neurosurg Focus 2011;31(5): E9 [A systematic review or a meta-analysis].

8. Micheli LJ, Wood R. Back pain in young athletes. Significant differences from adults in causes and patterns. Arch Pediatr Adolesc Med 1995;149(1):15–8.

9. Li Y, Hresko MT. Lumbar spine surgery in athletes: outcomes and return-to-play criteria. Clin Sports Med 2012;31(3):487–98.

10. Radcliff KE, Kalantar SB, Reitman CA. Surgical management of spondylolysis and spondylolisthesis in athletes: indications and return to play. Curr Sports Med Rep 2009;8(1):35–40.

11. Huang P, Anissipour A, McGee W, et al. Return-to-play recommendations after cervical, thoracic, and lumbar spine injuries: a comprehensive review. Sports Health 2016;8(1):19–25 [A systematic review or a meta-analysis].

12. Anakwenze OA, Namdari S, Auerbach JD, et al. Athletic performance outcomes following lumbar discectomy in professional basketball players. Spine 2010; 35(7):825–8.

13. Wang JC, Shapiro MS, Hatch JD, et al. The outcome of lumbar discectomy in elite athletes. Spine 1999;24(6):570–3.

14. Nair R, Kahlenberg CA, Hsu WK. Outcomes of lumbar discectomy in elite athletes: the need for high-level evidence. Clin Orthop Relat Res 2015;473(6): 1971–7 [A systematic review or a meta-analysis].

15. Overley SC, McAnany SJ, Andelman S, et al. Return to play in elite athletes after lumbar microdiscectomy: a meta-analysis. Spine (Phila Pa 1976) 2016;41(8): 713–8 [A systematic review or a meta-analysis].

16. Hsu WK, McCarthy KJ, Savage JW, et al. The Professional Athlete Spine Initiative: outcomes after lumbar disc herniation in 342 elite professional athletes. Spine J 2011;11(3):180–6.

17. Hsu WK. Performance-based outcomes following lumbar discectomy in professional athletes in the National Football League. Spine 2010;35(12):1247–51.

18. Weistroffer JK, Hsu WK. Return-to-play rates in National Football League linemen after treatment for lumbar disk herniation. Am J Sports Med 2011;39(3):632–6.

19. Savage JW, Hsu WK. Statistical performance in National Football League athletes after lumbar discectomy. Clin J Sport Med 2010;20(5):350–4.

20. Fleisig GS, Hsu WK, Fortenbaugh D, et al. Trunk axial rotation in baseball pitching and batting. Sports Biomech 2013;12(4):324–33.

21. Earhart JS, Roberts D, Roc G, et al. Effects of lumbar disk herniation on the careers of professional baseball players. Orthopedics 2012;35(1):43–9.

22. Minhas SV, Kester BS, Hsu WK. Outcomes after lumbar disc herniation in the National Basketball Association. Sports Health 2016;8(1):43–9.

23. Schroeder GD, McCarthy KJ, Micev AJ, et al. Performance-based outcomes after nonoperative treatment, discectomy, and/or fusion for a lumbar disc herniation in National Hockey League athletes. Am J Sports Med 2013;41(11):2604–8.

24. Watkins RG, Williams LA, Watkins RG 3rd. Microscopic lumbar discectomy results for 60 cases in professional and Olympic athletes. Spine J 2003;3(2):100–5.

25. Watkins RG, Hanna R, Chang D, et al. Return-to-play outcomes after microscopic lumbar diskectomy in professional athletes. Am J Sports Med 2012;40(11): 2530–5.

26. Burnett MG, Sonntag VK. Return to contact sports after spinal surgery. Neurosurg Focus 2006;21(4):E5.

27. Cahill KS, Dunn I, Gunnarsson T, et al. Lumbar microdiscectomy in pediatric patients: a large single-institution series. J Neurosurg Spine 2010;12(2):165–70.

28. Eck JC, Riley LH 3rd. Return to play after lumbar spine conditions and surgeries. Clin Sports Med 2004;23(3):367–79, viii.
29. Soler T, Calderon C. The prevalence of spondylolysis in the Spanish elite athlete. Am J Sports Med 2000;28(1):57–62.
30. Jackson DW, Wiltse LL, Cirincoine RJ. Spondylolysis in the female gymnast. Clin Orthop Relat Res 1976;(117):68–73.
31. Rossi F, Dragoni S. Lumbar spondylolysis: occurrence in competitive athletes. Updated achievements in a series of 390 cases. J Sports Med Phys Fitness 1990;30(4):450–2.
32. Bouras T, Korovessis P. Management of spondylolysis and low-grade spondylolisthesis in fine athletes. A comprehensive review. Eur J Orthop Surg Traumatol 2015;25(Suppl 1):S167–75 [A systematic review or a meta-analysis].
33. Menga EN, Kebaish KM, Jain A, et al. Clinical results and functional outcomes after direct intralaminar screw repair of spondylolysis. Spine 2014;39(1):104–10.
34. Snyder LA, Shufflebarger H, O'Brien MF, et al. Spondylolysis outcomes in adolescents after direct screw repair of the pars interarticularis. J Neurosurg Spine 2014;21(3):329–33.
35. Debnath UK, Freeman BJ, Gregory P, et al. Clinical outcome and return to sport after the surgical treatment of spondylolysis in young athletes. J Bone Joint Surg Br 2003;85(2):244–9.
36. Nozawa S, Shimizu K, Miyamoto K, et al. Repair of pars interarticularis defect by segmental wire fixation in young athletes with spondylolysis. Am J Sports Med 2003;31(3):359–64.
37. Durrani AA, Desai R, Chavanne A, et al. 125. Outcome of direct PARS repair in competitive athletes. Spine J 2008;8(Suppl 5):64S.
38. Sutton JH, Guin PD, Theiss SM. Acute lumbar spondylolysis in intercollegiate athletes. J Spinal Disord Tech 2012;25(8):422–5.
39. Gillis CC, Eichholz K, Thoman WJ, et al. A minimally invasive approach to defects of the pars interarticularis: Restoring function in competitive athletes. Clin Neurol Neurosurg 2015;139:29–34.
40. Rubery PT, Bradford DS. Athletic activity after spine surgery in children and adolescents: results of a survey. Spine 2002;27(4):423–7.
41. Abla AA, Maroon JC, Lochhead R, et al. Return to golf after spine surgery. J Neurosurg Spine 2011;14(1):23–30.
42. Siepe CJ, Wiechert K, Khattab MF, et al. Total lumbar disc replacement in athletes: clinical results, return to sport and athletic performance. Eur Spine J 2007;16(7):1001–13.
43. Tumialan LM, Ponton RP, Garvin A, et al. Arthroplasty in the military: a preliminary experience with ProDisc-C and ProDisc-L. Neurosurg Focus 2010;28(5):E18.
44. Fabricant PD, Admoni S, Green DW, et al. Return to athletic activity after posterior spinal fusion for adolescent idiopathic scoliosis: analysis of independent predictors. J Pediatr Orthop 2012;32(3):259–65.

Return to Play After Sports Hernia Surgery

Ho-Rim Choi, MD, Osama Elattar, MD, Vickie D. Dills, PT, DPT, Brian Busconi, MD*

KEYWORDS

- Sports hernia • Inguinal disruption • Surgical treatment • Return to sports

KEY POINTS

- Despite common presentation in the sports clinic, the definition, clinical characteristics, and treatment of sports hernia (SH) have not been fully understood.
- The clinical spectrum and treatment outcome of SH are reviewed.
- Details of nonoperative and postoperative rehabilitation processes are addressed in this article.

INTRODUCTION

SH is considered an overuse syndrome presenting with chronic lower abdomen and groin pain. Since Gilmore popularized the syndrome of groin disruption as Gilmore's groin in the early 1990s,[1] this condition has been named various terms, such as SH,[2–6] athletic pubalgia,[7] athletic hernia,[8] Gilmore's groin,[9,10] osteitis pubis, sportsman's hernia,[11,12] sportsmen's groin,[13] hockey groin syndrome,[14] symphysis syndrome,[15] and inguinal disruption.[16] In a recent consensus conference by the British Hernia Society in Manchester, United Kingdom, "inguinal disruption" was proposed as nomenclature for this condition.[17] Despite common presentation in the sports clinic, however, the definition, clinical characteristics, and treatment of SH have not been fully understood. The clinical spectrum of SH, with its treatment outcome and recovery process, is addressed in this article.

ANATOMY AND PATHOGENESIS

Fibers from the rectus abdominis, conjoint tendon (a fusion of the internal oblique and transversus abdominis), and external oblique merge to form the pubic aponeurosis. This pubic aponeurosis is confluent with the adductor and gracilis origin. SH is considered an injury to muscular and/or fascial attachments of these structures to the anterior pubis. There still is argument, however, regarding the exact anatomic area of disruption because even operative findings of SH repair is obscure.

Disclosure: Authors declare that they have no conflict of interest.
Department of Orthopaedic Surgery, University of Massachusetts, Hahnemann Campus, 281 Lincoln Street, Worcester, MA 01605, USA
* Corresponding author. Department of Orthopaedic Surgery, University of Massachusetts, Hahnemann Campus, 281 Lincoln Street, Worcester, MA 01605.
E-mail address: brian.busconi@umassmemorial.org

There are 2 possible explanations regarding the pathogenesis of SH.[7] One is muscle injury or disruption of structures listed previously. Investigators found the SH was associated with a torn external oblique aponeurosis, conjoined tendon, or abdominal wall abnormalities.[1,9,10,14,18,19] Another theory is a defect in the transversalis fascia, which forms the posterior wall of the inguinal canal, resulting in an occult hernia process.[4,8,20,21] In a retrospective analysis of 64 athletes of Australian rules footballers with chronic groin pain, the most common operative finding was a substantially deranged posterior wall of the inguinal canal.[21] Litwin and colleagues[7] concluded that a large tear or multiple small tears must be taking place to form an SH, involving 1 or several muscles in the region, which includes the external oblique aponeurosis, rectus abdominis, conjoined tendon/rectus abdominis interface, or individual muscles that form the conjoined tendon. They also explained that tears to any of these muscles could lead to the operative findings of attenuation, disruption, or retraction of the muscle, thereby weakening the boundaries of the posterior wall of the inguinal canal.[7] Theoretically, the shearing forces are more prominent in athletes with an imbalance between the strong adductor muscles of the thigh and the weak lower abdominal musculature. These forces place stress on the inguinal wall musculature, which ultimately leads to attenuation of local soft tissues.[3,22]

EPIDEMIOLOGY

The exact incidence of SH is not known, but several studies suggest that it is common in athletes with chronic groin pain.[3] Groin injuries account for approximately 1 in 20 athletic injuries, and groin pain accounts for 1 in 10 patient visits to sport medicine centers.[23] Injuries to the groin account for approximately 5% of all soccer injuries.[9,12]

SH occurs almost exclusively in men. The higher incidence of this condition in men may be explained by a greater level of participation of men in highly competitive sports.[24] An increasing number of female patients, however, are being diagnosed with this injury, ranging 10% to 15%.[25,26] Gender differences in pelvic anatomy, lower extremity alignment, and muscle activation may be another possible explanation for lower incidence of this condition in women.[27,28]

SH is also associated with professional athletes or high-performance school athletes. There is growing trend of occurrence, however, in recreational athletes.[7,24,28,29]

CLINICAL PRESENTATION

The hallmark symptom of SH is a complaint of gradually increasing activity-related lower abdominal and proximal adductor-related pain. The pain usually is relieved with rest but returns on resumption of sports.[3] Some patients may recall the specific event that initiated the pain; however, the onset is insidious in a majority of the patients.

The pain of lower abdomen or groin is often aggravated by certain movements, such as sudden acceleration, twisting, turning, and cutting or kicking. Soccer, hockey, ice hockey, American football, rugby, or Australian rules football players have a particularly high incidence.[5,7] Some patients complain of aggravated pain by sit-ups, coughing, or sneezing.[8,18,24,28] This pain may radiate to adductor region, perineum, inner thigh, and scrotum or testicular area.[18,25]

A cluster of 5 symptoms and signs are considered the most indicative of SH by Kachingwe and Grech[24]: (1) a subjective complaint of deep groin/lower abdominal pain; (2) pain that is exacerbated with sport-specific activities, such as sprinting, kicking, cutting, and/or sit-ups and is relieved with rest; (3) palpable tenderness over the pubic ramus at the insertion of the rectus abdominis and/or conjoined tendon; (4) pain with resisted hip adduction at 0°, 45°, and/or 90° of hip flexion; and (5) pain with resisted abdominal curl-up.[3,8,24,28–30]

Initial examination should be started with careful postural evaluation to find out any anterior pelvic tilt. The most common physical findings include localized tenderness at or just above pubic tubercle of the affected side where rectus abdominis attaches. The pain and tenderness are aggravated by resisted sit-ups. Patients usually do not have a detectable true inguinal hernia. Full examination of the hip joint, including range of motion (ROM), is required because joint motion—limiting disease, such as femoroacetabular impingement (FAI), is frequently associated with the HS. It is not uncommon that patients show combined adductor longus area pain and tenderness by resisted leg adduction or direct palpation. Positive pain and tenderness at adductor tendon origin may indicate requirement of additional procedure such as steroid injection or adductor tenotomy.[7,31]

DIAGNOSIS

Patients with groin pain may have a vast possible causes originating not only from orthopedic neuromuscular structures but also other physiologic system or medical subspecialties, such as general surgery, urology, or gynecology. Careful, thorough history and physical examination are key for accurate diagnosis.

The consensus meeting by the British Hernia Society[17] suggested criteria for diagnosis of inguinal disruption if at least 3 of the 5 clinical signs below are detectable: (1) pinpont tenderness over the pubic tubercle at the point of insertion of the conjoint tendon, (2) palpable tenderness over the deep inguinal ring, (3) pain and/or dilation of the external ring with no obvious hernia evident, (4) pain at the origin of the adductor longus tendon, and (5) dull, diffuse pain in the groin, often radiating to the perineum and inner thigh or across the midline.

IMAGING

No diagnostic imaging modality is sensitive and specific for the diagnosis of SH. Accordingly, imaging is useful primarily for excluding other pathologic conditions in the differential diagnosis.[2,3]

Plain Radiographs

Plain radiographs should include a well-aligned anteroposterior pelvis and a lateral view of the hip. These may demonstrate symphysis widening or bony erosion, pelvic avulsion fractures, apophyseal injuries, stress fractures, degenerative hip disease, underlying FAI, and dysplasia.

MRI

Many patients with SH frequently reveal nonspecific findings on MRI.[3] Therefore, it is useful for ruling out other causes of groin pain, such as stress fracture, avascular necrosis, or intra-articular hip abnormalities, including labral tears, articular cartilage lesions, or FAI.[8]

MRI is considered, however, the most appropriate diagnostic modality to evaluate SH because of its superiority of soft tissue evaluation. It can demonstrate partial tear or complete rupture of the rectus abdominis muscle or conjoint tendon fibers or bone marrow edema of pubic ramus (**Fig. 1**). Dedicated protocol designed to detect SH should be used when it is suspected clinically.[32,33] Albers and colleagues[34] obtained MRI of 32 athletes with pubalgia and found abnormalities in pubic symphysis (21/30); abdominal wall (27/30); groin musculature, including rectus abdominis (21/30); and

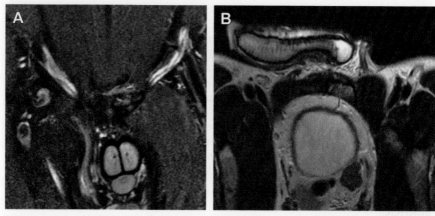

Fig. 1. (*A*) Coronal STIR and (*B*) oblique axial T2 images of pelvis MRI in a 22-year-old male patient show soft tissue signal change demonstrating rupture of left rectus abdominis muscle (*arrow*).

adductor muscle group (18/30). Zoga and colleagues[35] investigated MRI in 141 patients with groin pain and reported 68% of sensitivity and 100% specificity for rectus abdominis tendon injury and 86% sensitivity and 89% of specificity for adductor tendon injury.

Ultrasound

Dynamic high-resolution ultrasound can be a useful noninvasive modality for evaluating SH as the patient actively strains during the procedure. Orchard and colleagues[36] investigated 35 professional Australian footballers and found that dynamic ultrasound examination was able to detect inguinal canal posterior wall deficiency in 21 of 35 patients. Advantages of ultrasound examination are that it is a less expensive than MRI, noninvasive modality but a disadvantage is that it is highly operator dependent with variable reproducibility.[8]

DIFFERENTIAL DIAGNOSIS

There are several causes of chronic lower abdomen and groin pain that need to be differentiated from SH: disorders of the hip joint, injury to muscles of the thigh or abdominal wall, and even genitourinary or intra-abdominal disease. Before making a diagnosis of SH, many of these conditions should be differentiated by careful history, physical examination, and imaging studies[37] (**Box 1**).

Femoroacetabular Impingement

FAI is a condition that proximal femoral neck abuts acetabulum with ROM, especially in flexion. Patients usually present with activity-related groin or hip pain with limited hip flexion and internal rotation. Physical examination typically shows groin pain, which is elicited by anterior impingement test. Plain radiographs show decreased head-to-neck ratio, aspherical femoral head, or overhanging of acetabular rim. MRI is the best modality to evaluate associated lesion of acetabular labrum and articular cartilage. Surgical correction of bony deformity of cam or/and pincer combined with labral repair is indicated for symptomatic patients who are not responsive to conservative management.

Box 1
Differential diagnosis for groin pain

Hip joint
- Acetabular labral tear
- FAI
- Adductor injury
- Osteoarthritis
- Avascular necrosis
- Femoral neck stress fracture

Muscle and tendon
- Sports hernia
- Adductor strain/tendinitis
- Rectus femoris strain/tear
- Iliopsoas strain/tendinitis

Surrounding bone lesion
- Osteitis pubis
- Pubic ramus fracture
- Avulsion fracture: avulsion anterior superior iliac spine, avulsion anterior inferior iliac spine

Intra-abdominal
- Endometriosis
- Ovarian cystic disease
- Pelvic inflammatory disease
- Crohn disease

Abdominal hernia
- Inguinal hernia
- Femoral hernia

Genitourinary
- Epididymitis
- Prostatitis
- Testicular tumors
- Urethritis

Adductor Strain

Pulled groin commonly occurs in 10% to 30% of soccer and hockey players by strong eccentric contraction of adductors during play. Pain develops immediately after an acute injury and many patients shows pain and decreased muscle strength with resisted leg adduction. MRI shows adductor muscle injury, such as muscle edema, hemorrhage, or occasional bony avulsion in juvenile players. Nonoperative management followed by rehabilitation and gradual return to sports is suggested.

Osteitis Pubis

Osteitis pubic is an inflammation of the pubic symphysis caused by repetitive micro-trauma by sports, such as soccer, hockey, football and running involving kicking/adduction/abduction. Symptom is vague, ill-defined pain at anterior pelvis region. The unique physical finding is localized tenderness directly over the pubis symphysis. Plain radiographs are frequently show osteolytic pubis with bony erosion. This is a self-limiting process and may take several months to resolve by nonoperative management.

TREATMENT

In general, many SH patients visit orthopedic sports clinics and then undergo surgery by hernia surgeons after consultation with general surgery. Physiotherapy shares an important role for both nonoperative and postoperative treatment of rehabilitation. Radiology also performs a critical role to obtain detail information of anatomic structure based on imaging studies. Therefore, a multidisciplinary therapeutic approach is necessary for best outcome. In addition, multiple factors should be addressed when treatment decisions are made: degree of limitation and athletes' ability to participate in the sports, sports seasons and upcoming athletic events, response to prior treatment modalities, and level of athletes.[38]

Nonsurgical Treatment

It is agreed that surgery is not always indicated and nonoperative management should be attempted for all athletes as the first line of treatment if an athlete is in season and able to function at a high level despite pain: 4-week to 8-week trial of rest, oral analgesics and anti-inflammatory medications, steroid injection to the rectus abdominis insertion or the adductor longus origin, and physical therapy.[7,17,38]

Physical therapy concentrates on stretching/strengthening, core stabilization, postural retraining, and restoration of balance to the abdominal wall, hip, and pelvis muscles. Aggressive stretching and attempts at improving ROM are not recommended because they can result in increased hip pain with underlying hip pathology, such as labral lesion or FAI.[5,29] Larson and Lohnes[39] outlined a 4-phase rehabilitation protocol for athletes with chronic groin pain. Phase 1 (weeks 1 and 2) focuses on massage and stretching. Phase 2 (weeks 3 and 4) emphasizes abdominal muscle strengthening. In phase 3 (week 5), functional activities, including running, are initiated. In phase 4 (week 6), the athlete returns to sport-specific activities.[39] At approximately 10 weeks to 12 weeks after the start of conservative treatment and when the athlete is pain-free, return to sports competition is generally attempted.

Ultrasound-guided steroid injection into the rectus abdominis insertion site, conjoined tendon, or adductor tendon can be a useful nonoperative management option during the season if an athlete wants to keep playing. In the authors' institute, in-season or preseason nonoperative management starts with 1 weeks to 2 weeks trial of rest with selective steroid or platelet-rich plasma injections to the rectus abdominis insertion and/or the adductor longus origin. At the completion of the rest period, an exercise program emphasizing strengthening, soft tissue and joint mobilization, and dynamic stability exercises is followed with cardiovascular training (**Table 1**).

In general, however, SH is known to be poorly responsive to nonoperative treatment and there are few data evaluating the efficacy of nonoperative treatment.[2,3,8,12,15,40] Paajanen and colleagues[41] performed a randomized, prospective comparative study between 30 operative versus 30 physiotherapy for sportsman's hernia and demonstrated that operative repair was more effective than nonoperative treatment to

Table 1
Rehabilitation protocol for nonoperative management with/without corticosteroid injection

In-Season	Week	Postseason
• Rest (injected) structures	1–2	• Rest (injected) structures

• ROM lumbar and bilateral hip joints
• Gluteal muscle and anterior pelvis
stabilization
  ○ Hip hikes
  ○ Abdominal bracing in hook lying
  ○ Front and side planks
  ○ Quadruped alternating upper and
    lower extremity on compliant and
    noncompliant surfaces
• Stationary bike without resistance
	3	• ROM lumbar and bilateral hip joints
		• Gluteal muscle and anterior pelvis
		stabilization
		  ○ Hip hikes
		  ○ Abdominal bracing in hook lying
		  ○ Front and side planks
		  ○ Quadruped alternating upper and
		    lower extremity on compliant and
		    noncompliant surfaces
		• Stationary bike without resistance

• Continue week 3 exercises • Flexion only straight leg raises; progress to multiplane • Supine hip extension with knee at 0 and 90° • Single-leg balance exercises • Bridging • Wall squats at 45°–90°	4	• Continue week 3 exercises • Flexion only straight leg raises; progress to multiplane • Supine hip extension with knee at 0 and 90° • Single-leg balance exercises • Bridging • Wall squats at 45°–90°
• Resistance walking, pushing, pulling • Return-to-running/jumping program (single plane) • Box jumps • Tilt board, agility ladder, and BOSU drills	5	• Continue weeks 3–4 exercises
• Progress core stabilization exercises • Increase resistive exercise as tolerated • Initiate sport-specific exercise program	6	• Continue weeks 3–4 exercises
• Continue with progressive sport- specific program • Gradual return to sport through pro- gressive practice participation	7–8	• Progress core stabilization exercises • Increase resistive exercise as tolerated • Initiate sport-specific exercise program
• Return to play	9	• Gradual return to sport through pro- gressive practice participation

decrease chronic groin pain after 1 month and up to 12 months of follow-up; 27 of 30 athletes (90%) who underwent operation returned to sports activities after 3 months of convalescence compared with 8 (27%) of the 30 athletes in the nonoperative group.[41] On the other hand, Kachingwe and Grech[24] suggested that conservative management, including manual therapy, could be a viable option in the management of athletes with an athletic pubalgia based on their decision making.[24]

Surgical Treatment

Surgical exploration and repair should be considered when nonoperative treatment has failed and the athlete continues to experience pain and disability during the season. Higher-level athletes who completed the season but struggled with chronic pain might be considered for surgery during off season. A variety of surgical techniques have been reported in the literature, including open repair of the rectus abdominis, external oblique, transversus abdominis or transversalis fascia, repairs with mesh reinforcement, laparoscopic repairs, miniopen repairs, and broad pelvic floor repairs with or without adductor releases.

Open surgeries

Gilmore[9] reported repair of torn external oblique aponeurosis, conjoined tendon, and dehiscence between conjoined tendon and inguinal ligaments for more than 1000 soccer players. The surgery was successful in 97% of cases with average player return to league football within 6 weeks.[9] Hackney[4] reported excellent results of surgical repair of the posterior inguinal wall for SH; 14 of 15 patients (87%) could successfully return to full sporting activity after their postoperative protocol: stretching and non–weight-bearing exercise, such as swimming or cycling after 3 weeks, and running at 4 to 5 weeks, daily training at 6 weeks.[4] Meyers and colleagues[28] reported outcome of the pelvic floor repair in 175 high-performance athletes, which involved open broad surgical reattachment of the inferolateral edge of the rectus abdominis muscle with its fascial investment to the pubis and adjacent anterior ligaments with/without adductor longus release.[19,28] They reported 88% of patients were performing at or above their preinjury levels of performance at 3 months after surgery and 96% at 6 months. Jans and colleagues[42] analyzed outcome of 241 male athletes of chronic sportsman's hernia. They underwent surgical intervention with reinforcement of the posterior inguinal wall and tenotomy of the adductors. More than 90% of 162 athletes could achieve satisfactory results.[42] Ahumada and colleagues[29] reported 12 patients with athletic pubalgia who underwent open inguinal repair, with 9 reinforced with mesh. Results were 83.3% excellent and 16.7% satisfactory, and all returned to sports by median 4 months of follow-up.[29] In the authors' institute, open suture repair is preferred focusing on (1) repair and retensioning of the rectus abdominis to the pubis and broadening of its insertion, (2) stabilization of the conjoined tendon/rectus abdominis interface, and (3) reinforcement of the posterior wall of the inguinal canal.[7]

Surgery is performed by a general surgeon with a special interest in abdominal wall disorders and an orthopedic sports medicine specialist together as a multidisciplinary team approach. A short groin incision along skin crease is made and external oblique muscle is exposed through subcutaneous fat dissection. This muscle is opened in the direction of its fibers and separated from underlying structures. The spermatic cord is retracted inferiorly to expose the posterior wall of the inguinal canal. Attenuation and bulging of the posterior wall or disruption of the rectus abdominis or conjoined tendon is repaired at this point (**Fig. 2**A). At the beginning of the repair, the pubic tubercle is roughened with electrocautery to create an inflammatory surface and the lateral edge of rectus is brought down to the periosteum of the tubercle with 1 or 2 stitches using Orthocord (DePuy Orthopaedics, Warsaw, Indiana). The edge of rectus is brought down to the Cooper ligament with 1 stitch, followed by 1 interrupted suture approximating the conjoined tendon/rectus abdominis interface with the shelving portion of the ilioinguinal ligament. At this point, 1 or 2 reinforcing stitches extend laterally, pulling conjoined tendon to shelving portion (**Fig. 2**B). All nerves are preserved. The cord is then dropped back into position, and the external oblique aponeurosis closed as well as the skin and subcutaneous tissues.[7] If the adductor longus symptom is involved, it can either be injected with steroid or platelet-rich plasma, or tendon release/lengthening is performed at the time of surgery.

Laparoscopic surgeries or minimal repair

Laparoscopic treatment offers the potential advantage of a more rapid recovery and return to sport than does open hernia repair. Genitsaris and colleagues[20] reviewed 131 athletes with chronic groin pain who underwent laparoscopic repair of deficiency

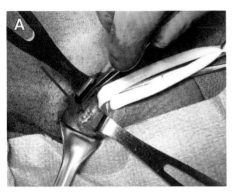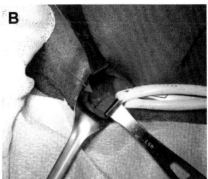

Fig. 2. A 25-year-old professional football player shows (*A*) attenuated rectus abdominis muscle insertion to the pubic tubercle (*arrow*). (*B*) Rectus abdonimis was retensioned with reinforcement of posterior inguinal wall (*arrow*).

of the posterior inguinal wall. All patients were able to back to full sporting activities within 2 to 3 weeks and there was only 1 recurrence (0.76%) after a mean follow-up of 5 years.[20] Rossidis and colleagues[43] reported 100% successful return to full sports-related activity of 54 athlete patients treated by laparoscopic extraperitoneal inguinal hernia repair with synthetic mesh combined with ipsilateral adductor longus tenotomy. All patients were able to return to full sports-related activity in 24 days (range 21–28 days).[43] van Veen and colleagues[30] reported that 55 professional and semiprofessional sportsmen with chronic groin pain were treated by endoscopic total extraperitoneal mesh placement, and all the athletes could return to their normal sports level within 3 months after the operation.[30] In a comparative study between open versus laparoscopic repairs for groin disruption, the open repairs could restart full-contact training at a median 5 weeks (range 1–6) versus 3 weeks (range 1–9) for the laparoscopic repairs.[44]

On the other hand, Economopoulos and colleagues[45] compared the outcome of 14 modified Bassini repairs and 14 minimal repair techniques. They found that the patients in the minimal repair group returned to sports earlier (5.6 weeks vs 25.8 weeks) and higher success rates of returning to sports at their preinjury level of play (13/14 vs 9/14).

Concurrent Management of Associated Pathology

Because there is increasing awareness of an association between ROM-limiting hip disorders, such as FAI or intra-articular hip pathology and SH in athletes, it is important to consider concurrent management of those lesions.[37,46,47] Hammoud and colleagues[46] reported that 39% of patients who underwent arthroscopic surgery for symptomatic FAI resolved athletic pubalgia symptoms and emphasized drawing attention to the overlap of these 2 diagnoses.[46] Larson and colleagues[37] evaluated follow-up outcome of 37 hips diagnosed with both symptomatic athletic pubalgia and symptomatic intra-articular hip joint pathology. They found surgical management of both disorders concurrently or in a staged manner led to improved postoperative outcome scoring and an unrestricted return to sporting activity in 89% of hips, whereas the hips only addressed either the athletic pubalgia or intra-articular hip pathology showed suboptimal outcomes.[37]

In addition, treatment of a contracted or overdeveloped adductor muscle also need to be addressed. Investigators recommend adductor tenotomy combined with hernia repair when symptomatic adductor abnormality cannot be corrected preoperatively.[29,31,43] The improvement of adductor pain after SH repair suggests that adductor tendinitis may be a secondary phenomenon to the SH or initial injury. If the theory regarding an imbalance between the strong adductors and weak abdominal muscles is true, then additional procedure, such as adductor release, adductor tendon injection, or osteoplasty for FAI, may be a reasonable measurement to decrease symptoms and protect the pelvic floor procedure.[7,8]

RETURN TO SPORTS AFTER SURGERY

Both nonoperative and postoperative treatment options share the goal of returning the athlete back to pain-free activity. There is little research available, however, to reference for rehabilitation guidelines and creation of therapeutic plan in regard to timing back to sports activities after surgery or nonoperative management.[48]

The consensus meeting by the British Hernia Society[17] suggested that appropriate preoperative and postoperative care should allow a full return to activity within 4 weeks to 8 weeks from the date of surgery.[17] They also emphasized that close liaison between the treating clinicians and the physiotherapy team is required for the preoperative and postoperative rehabilitation. Litwin and colleagues[7] reported their postoperative rehabilitation and recovery process after open reattachment of the rectus and reinforcement of the posterior wall of the inguinal canal. The patient is allowed weight bearing as tolerated with relative rest for the first 10 days and gentle hip ROM. Closed-chain lower extremity exercises are permitted for the next 2 weeks. At approximately week 4, light abdominal core exercises are added, and at approximately week 5, sport-specific activity is advanced as tolerated. Full return to sport is at approximately 6 weeks. Gilmore[9] analyzed groin pain in soccer athletes and suggested intensive groin disruption rehabilitation program after surgical repair: week 1, walk 2 times a day; week 2, jog in straight lines and start adductor exercises; week 3, run in straight lines and increase adductor exercises; and week 4, sprint and start kicking; may play. The average player was reported to be able to return to league football within 6 weeks.[9] Biedert and colleagues[15] treated 24 athletes of chronic symphysis syndrome by spreading of the lateral border of the sheath of the rectus abdominis muscle or reconstruction of the muscle together with an epimysial adductor release. The patients started postoperative physical therapy and rehabilitation on the first day after surgery with immediate isometric contractions of the abdominal and adductor muscles under physical therapy control. Full training was allowed after 6 weeks to 8 weeks when the athlete was completely pain-free, and competition was allowed after 10 to 12 weeks. Full sports activity was noted in 23 of 24 athletes at a mean of 6.6 years posttreatment.[15] Hemingway and colleagues[49] described a 6-week post–open SH repair rehabilitation program, which involved both attending physiotherapy once a week and a standardized home exercise program: week 1, isometric abdominals and hip exercises, walk increased by 5 min/d, and stairs; week 2: active exercises for hips, transverse and oblique abdominals, and exercise bike; week 3: flexibility work, Thera-Band hip exercises, transverse and oblique abdominals, jogging, and swimming; week 4: running forward, progressing to abdominal work, and low upper body weights; week 5: sprinting, running in all directions, light ball skills, kicking, abdominals, and gradual return to training; and week 6: full training, match play, and return to play. They could achieve the most significant improvement of abdominal obliques strength by rehabilitation.

In the authors' institute, athletes are recommended to rest for 1 week to 2 weeks after surgery, anticipating wound healing and pain control. Normal passive hip ROM with isometric abdominal and hip exercises is restored this phase (phase I) (**Box 2**).

Box 2
Rehabilitation protocol after surgical repair of sports hernia (phase I)

Day 1 through week 2: rest, tendinous healing and remodeling

Goals:

- Protect surgical site
- Wound care
- Pain control
- Edema reduction
- Improve soft tissue flexibility
- Restore normal passive hip ROM
- Educate patient on precautions, restrictions, and plan of care

Rehabilitation

- Gentle, passive ROM to bilateral hip joints; avoid painful end ranges and excessive hip abduction and extension, which stress the surgical sites
- Joint mobilization of the lumbar spine grades II–III for pain control and lumbar mobility
  ○ Hip anterior glide mobilization in supine
  ○ Hip posterior glide mobilization in supine
  ○ Central lumbar mobilization
  ○ Anterior ilium rotation mobilization
  ○ Posterior ilium rotation mobilization
- Soft tissue mobilization of lumbar paraspinal muscles
- Scar mobilization as soon as incision sutures are removed; deep transverse friction massage, instrument assisted soft tissue mobilization
- Stationary bike without resistance, avoid trunk hyperextension
- Patient education for pelvic neutral in sitting and standing
- Restore normal walking gait patterns
- Avoid activities, which increase intra-abdominal pressure
- No lifting or other activities that increase abdominal pressures
- Ice 15 minutes every 2 to 4 hours for the first 24 to 48 hours

---

Progressive exercise is performed focusing on hip ROM, core strengthening, postural exercise, and improving biomechanics in 3 weeks to 4 weeks (phase II) (**Box 3**). Sport-specific movements with plyometric exercise and agility drill starts in 5 weeks to 8 weeks after surgery to return to sports (phase III) (**Box 4**).

Success rates to return to sports have been reported ranging from 80% to 100%.[4,5,13,20,26,28,50–52] According to a systematic literature review, overall postsurgical recovery time based on return-to-sports activity for patients who underwent open repair was 17.7 weeks compared with 6.1 weeks for laparoscopic repairs.[2] It seems there are some common concepts among most surgeons regarding timing back-to-sports activities after surgery of SH, despite that direct comparison of these outcomes is difficult because of different patient populations and a variety of surgical techniques. In general, most athletes return to sports participation within 2 to 6 weeks after laparoscopic repair and within 1 to 6 months after open repair.[3,28,29]

Box 3
Rehabilitation protocol after surgical repair of sports hernia (phase II)

Weeks 3 to 4: continue to increase hip ROM, core strength, improve biomechanics

Goals

- Target strengthening and neuromuscular re-education with a focus on timing and recruitment patterns during functional movements
- Identify muscle imbalances, postural deviations, and muscular compensations
- Advance core strength and stability
- Advance cardiovascular training

Rehabilitation: monitor patient pain levels and progress as tolerated

- Stretching to increase and restore flexibility of all lower extremity muscle groups including hamstrings, adductors, gluteal muscles, hip flexors, ankle dorsiflexors, and quadriceps
- Core strengthening/core stability exercises with emphasis on gluteus medius, gluteus maximus, TA, and multifidus
  - Isometric abdominals with focus on TA and obliques to facilitate TA recruitment; start in supine and progress to quadruped, kneeling and half-kneeling positions
  - Dead bugs
  - Glute bridges progressing to glute bridges with resistance bands
  - Front and side planks
  - Double-leg and single-leg bridging
  - Rocker board drills
- Progressive resistive exercises
  - Straight leg raises for hip flexors
  - Wall squats for hamstrings and quadriceps
  - Heel raises for gastroc/soleus
  - Lateral band walks for hip abductors; maintain lumbar neutral control
  - PNF diagonals with sport cord
  - Crossband core work initiated in supine and progressed to standing
- Straight plane motion in weight bearing
  - Forward lunges (avoid deep lunges)
  - Single-leg dead lifts
  - Leg presses
  - Wall slides at less than 90° progressing to 90° while extending hold times
  - Step-ups and step-downs; focus on eccentric quad control and proper pelvic alignment
- Proprioceptive training
  - Single-leg balance exercise to include cone taps, single-leg ball toss
  - Exercises on unstable, noncompliant surfaces, such as foam pads, tilt board, BOSU ball
  - Balance reach exercises with both lower and upper extremities
  - Single and multiplane wobble board drills
- Cardiovascular training
  - Continue with seated or recumbent bike adding resistance in pain-free intensities; seated recruits gluteals more than the recumbent bike
  - Elliptical (pain-free)
  - Stable surface or treadmill walking

Abbreviations: PNF, proprioceptive neuromascular facilitation; TA, transversus abdominis.

SUMMARY

Groin pain can be presented as a complex clinical feature. It may be related to injury of the soft tissue, bone, or joints from an orthopedic, neurologic, urologic, or general surgical issue, which essentially requires multidisciplinary approach. Proper evaluation by

Box 4
Rehabilitation protocol after surgical repair of sports hernia (phase III)

Weeks 5 to 8: return-to-sports/plyometric exercises

Goals

- Prescribe sport-specific movements and speeds to prepare and strengthen the involved tissue for the forced couples created during sport-specific movements
- Progress to running on uneven surfaces progressing to an intensity required for specific sport
- Return to full play without pain

Rehabilitation: exercise in all 3 planes of motion. Implement return-to-running and sport-specific activities in both open and closed kinetic chain. Monitor patient pain levels and progress as tolerated.

- Core strengthening/core stability exercises
  - 3-Way planks
  - Prone physioball walkouts
  - Dynamic planks
  - Resisted core exercise using medicine balls, sports cords, weights
  - Advanced cross-band resisted core exercises

- Triplane weight-bearing exercises
  - Forward and lateral lunges
  - TRX/Rip 60 double-leg and single-leg squats
  - Resisted band ambulation forward, backward and lateral
  - Speed skaters progressing to resisted speed skaters
  - Slide board drills

- Proprioceptive training
  - Sport cord arcs
  - Sport forward and backward shuffles
  - Single-leg ladder drills
  - Single-leg BOSU drills

- Cardiovascular training
  - Return to running on even, flat ground
  - Line jumps/box jumps
  - Progress to running on uneven surfaces progressing to an intensity required for specific sport
  - Sport-specific sprinting, endurance running, changes in direction
  - Ladder drills
  - High knees, butt kicks, bounding, high skipping, bear crawls

- Plyometric exercises
  - BOSU drills
  - Box jumps
  - Medicine ball tosses/lunges
  - Weighted rope drills
  - Cone drills

- Agility drills
  - Straight running at a steady pace, 20 to 30 minutes
  - High knee drills
  - Lateral running in crouched position
  - Backward running
  - Vertical jumping
  - Stair climbing
  - Carioca drills
  - Line touch drills
  - Figure-8 running
  - Run and cut

- Sport-specific drills to include
  - Court sports: vertical leaping, box out drills, initiate plant/pivot, change direction, stop/start
  - Soccer: cone dribbling, initiate plant/pivot, change directions, stop/start, increase training/sprinting
  - Hockey: slide board drills with and without stick, initiate start/stop, skating practice drills with team, shooting
  - Football: plant/pivot, change directions, short sprints, long sprints, lateral bounds, squat jumps, crossover drills

careful history and meticulous physical examination is the first step for an accurate diagnosis. Surgical intervention, both open and laparoscopic, is frequently required, leading to excellent results in most reported studies. Well-designed research studies are warranted to better understand the pathogenesis and short-term and long-term outcomes based on therapeutic measurement and to establish most effective rehabilitation and preventive training protocol.

REFERENCES

1. Gilmore J. Gilmore's groin: ten years experience of groin disruption- a previously unsolved problem in sportsmen. Sports Med Soft Tissue Trauma 1991;1(3):12–4.
2. Caudill P, Nyland J, Smith C, et al. Sports hernias: a systematic literature review. Br J Sports Med 2008;42(12):954–64.
3. Farber AJ, Wilckens JH. Sports hernia: diagnosis and therapeutic approach. J Am Acad Orthop Surg 2007;15(8):507–14.
4. Hackney RG. The sports hernia: a cause of chronic groin pain. Br J Sports Med 1993;27(1):58–62.
5. Larson CM. Sports hernia/athletic pubalgia: evaluation and management. Sports Health 2014;6(2):139–44.
6. Minnich JM, Hanks JB, Muschaweck U, et al. Sports hernia: diagnosis and treatment highlighting a minimal repair surgical technique. Am J Sports Med 2011;39(6):1341–9.
7. Litwin DE, Sneider EB, McEnaney PM, et al. Athletic pubalgia (sports hernia). Clin Sports Med 2011;30(2):417–34.
8. Swan KG Jr, Wolcott M. The athletic hernia: a systematic review. Clin Orthop Relat Res 2007;455:78–87.
9. Gilmore J. Groin pain in the soccer athlete: fact, fiction, and treatment. Clin Sports Med 1998;17(4):787–93, vii.
10. Williams P, Foster ME. 'Gilmore's groin'–or is it? Br J Sports Med 1995;29(3):206–8.
11. Fon LJ, Spence RA. Sportsman's hernia. Br J Surg 2000;87(5):545–52.
12. Moeller JL. Sportsman's hernia. Curr Sports Med Rep 2007;6(2):111–4.
13. Muschaweck U, Berger L. Minimal Repair technique of sportsmen's groin: an innovative open-suture repair to treat chronic inguinal pain. Hernia 2010;14(1):27–33.
14. Irshad K, Feldman LS, Lavoie C, et al. Operative management of "hockey groin syndrome": 12 years of experience in National Hockey League players. Surgery 2001;130(4):759–64 [discussion: 64–6].
15. Biedert RM, Warnke K, Meyer S. Symphysis syndrome in athletes: surgical treatment for chronic lower abdominal, groin, and adductor pain in athletes. Clin J Sport Med 2003;13(5):278–84.

16. Sheen AJ, Iqbal Z. Contemporary management of 'Inguinal disruption' in the sportsman's groin. BMC Sports Sci Med Rehabil 2014;6:39.

17. Sheen AJ, Stephenson BM, Lloyd DM, et al. 'Treatment of the sportsman's groin': British Hernia Society's 2014 position statement based on the Manchester Consensus Conference. Br J Sports Med 2014;48(14):1079–87.

18. Nam A, Brody F. Management and therapy for sports hernia. J Am Coll Surg 2008;206(1):154–64.

19. Taylor DC, Meyers WC, Moylan JA, et al. Abdominal musculature abnormalities as a cause of groin pain in athletes. Inguinal hernias and pubalgia. Am J Sports Med 1991;19(3):239–42.

20. Genitsaris M, Goulimaris I, Sikas N. Laparoscopic repair of groin pain in athletes. Am J Sports Med 2004;32(5):1238–42.

21. Polglase AL, Frydman GM, Farmer KC. Inguinal surgery for debilitating chronic groin pain in athletes. Med J Aust 1991;155(10):674–7.

22. LeBlanc KE, LeBlanc KA. Groin pain in athletes. Hernia 2003;7(2):68–71.

23. Suarez JC, Ely EE, Mutnal AB, et al. Comprehensive approach to the evaluation of groin pain. J Am Acad Orthop Surg 2013;21(9):558–70.

24. Kachingwe AF, Grech S. Proposed algorithm for the management of athletes with athletic pubalgia (sports hernia): a case series. J Orthop Sports Phys Ther 2008; 38(12):768–81.

25. Garvey JF, Read JW, Turner A. Sportsman hernia: what can we do? Hernia 2010; 14(1):17–25.

26. Meyers WC, McKechnie A, Philippon MJ, et al. Experience with "sports hernia" spanning two decades. Ann Surg 2008;248(4):656–65.

27. Brophy RH, Backus S, Kraszewski AP, et al. Differences between sexes in lower extremity alignment and muscle activation during soccer kick. J Bone Joint Surg Am 2010;92(11):2050–8.

28. Meyers WC, Foley DP, Garrett WE, et al. Management of severe lower abdominal or inguinal pain in high-performance athletes. PAIN (Performing Athletes with Abdominal or Inguinal Neuromuscular Pain Study Group). Am J Sports Med 2000;28(1):2–8.

29. Ahumada LA, Ashruf S, Espinosa-de-los-Monteros A, et al. Athletic pubalgia: definition and surgical treatment. Ann Plast Surg 2005;55(4):393–6.

30. van Veen RN, de Baat P, Heijboer MP, et al. Successful endoscopic treatment of chronic groin pain in athletes. Surg Endosc 2007;21(2):189–93.

31. Van Der Donckt K, Steenbrugge F, Van Den Abbeele K, et al. Bassini's hernial repair and adductor longus tenotomy in the treatment of chronic groin pain in athletes. Acta Orthop Belg 2003;69(1):35–41.

32. Omar IM, Zoga AC, Kavanagh EC, et al. Athletic pubalgia and "sports hernia": optimal MR imaging technique and findings. Radiographics 2008;28(5):1415–38.

33. Palisch A, Zoga AC, Meyers WC. Imaging of athletic pubalgia and core muscle injuries: clinical and therapeutic correlations. Clin Sports Med 2013;32(3):427–47.

34. Albers SL, Spritzer CE, Garrett WE Jr, et al. MR findings in athletes with pubalgia. Skeletal Radiol 2001;30(5):270–7.

35. Zoga AC, Kavanagh EC, Omar IM, et al. Athletic pubalgia and the "sports hernia": MR imaging findings. Radiology 2008;247(3):797–807.

36. Orchard JW, Read JW, Neophyton J, et al. Groin pain associated with ultrasound finding of inguinal canal posterior wall deficiency in Australian Rules footballers. Br J Sports Med 1998;32(2):134–9.

37. Larson CM, Pierce BR, Giveans MR. Treatment of athletes with symptomatic intra-articular hip pathology and athletic pubalgia/sports hernia: a case series. Arthroscopy 2011;27(6):768–75.

38. Larson CM, Birmingham PM, Oliver SM. Athletic Publagia. In: Miller MD, Thompson SR, editors. DeLee & Drez's orthopaedic sports medicine. 4th edition. Saunders; 2014. p. 966–74, 74.e2.

39. Larson CM, Lohnes JH. Surgical management of athletic publagia. Oper Tech Sports Med 2002;10:228–32.

40. Holmich P, Uhrskou P, Ulnits L, et al. Effectiveness of active physical training as treatment for long-standing adductor-related groin pain in athletes: randomised trial. Lancet 1999;353(9151):439–43.

41. Paajanen H, Brinck T, Hermunen H, et al. Laparoscopic surgery for chronic groin pain in athletes is more effective than nonoperative treatment: a randomized clinical trial with magnetic resonance imaging of 60 patients with sportsman's hernia (athletic pubalgia). Surgery 2011;150(1):99–107.

42. Jans C, Messaoudi N, Pauli S, et al. Results of surgical treatment of athletes with sportsman's hernia. Acta Orthop Belg 2012;78(1):35–40.

43. Rossidis G, Perry A, Abbas H, et al. Laparoscopic hernia repair with adductor tenotomy for athletic pubalgia: an established procedure for an obscure entity. Surg Endosc 2015;29(2):381–6.

44. Ingoldby CJ. Laparoscopic and conventional repair of groin disruption in sportsmen. Br J Surg 1997;84(2):213–5.

45. Economopoulos KJ, Milewski MD, Hanks JB, et al. Sports hernia treatment: modified bassini versus minimal repair. Sports Health 2013;5(5):463–9.

46. Hammoud S, Bedi A, Magennis E, et al. High incidence of athletic pubalgia symptoms in professional athletes with symptomatic femoroacetabular impingement. Arthroscopy 2012;28(10):1388–95.

47. Munegato D, Bigoni M, Gridavilla G, et al. Sports hernia and femoroacetabular impingement in athletes: a systematic review. World J Clin Cases 2015;3(9):823–30.

48. Ellsworth AA, Zoland MP, Tyler TF. Athletic pubalgia and associated rehabilitation. Int J Sports Phys Ther 2014;9(6):774–84.

49. Hemingway AE, Herrington L, Blower AL. Changes in muscle strength and pain in response to surgical repair of posterior abdominal wall disruption followed by rehabilitation. Br J Sports Med 2003;37(1):54–8.

50. Brannigan AE, Kerin MJ, McEntee GP. Gilmore's groin repair in athletes. J Orthop Sports Phys Ther 2000;30(6):329–32.

51. Brown RA, Mascia A, Kinnear DG, et al. An 18-year review of sports groin injuries in the elite hockey player: clinical presentation, new diagnostic imaging, treatment, and results. Clin J Sport Med 2008;18(3):221–6.

52. Kluin J, den Hoed PT, van Linschoten R, et al. Endoscopic evaluation and treatment of groin pain in the athlete. Am J Sports Med 2004;32(4):944–9.

Return to Play Following Hip Arthroscopy

Simon Lee, MD, MPH[a], Andrew Kuhn, BA[b], Pete Draovitch, PT, MS, ATC, CSCS, SCS[c], Asheesh Bedi, MD[d],*

KEYWORDS

- Hip • Hip arthroscopy • Femoroacetabular impingement • Labral tear • Sport
- Return to play

KEY POINTS

- Femoroacetabular impingement (FAI) may be particularly disabling to the high-demand athlete, especially those with significant cutting and pivoting requirements.
- Awareness of varying demographics among different groups of athletes are important to identify the individual needs of patients when considering preventive, nonoperative, or surgical management options.
- Return to play is high with professional, amateur, adolescent athletes, as well as athletes undergoing concomitant microfracture and labral reconstruction techniques.
- Important considerations include the ability to achieve the diagnosis in a timely manner and to exercise caution in older athletes with presence of preexisting osteoarthritis or diminished joint space, as the literature demonstrates suboptimal outcomes in these populations.

INTRODUCTION

Improvements in diagnostic tools and our awareness has led to a significant increase in the recognition and treatment of symptomatic pathologies in the young, nonarthritic hip. Femoroacetabular impingement (FAI) is the most common cause of prearthritic pain and secondary chondro-labral pathology in the nondysplastic hip. The structural deformities of FAI most commonly reflect a loss of femoral head-neck offset (cam-type lesion), as well as focal or global acetabular over coverage (pincer-type lesion). Most

[a] University of Michigan Health System, 1500 East Medical Center Drive, TC2912, Ann Arbor, MI 48109-5328, USA; [b] Domino's Farms – MedSport, University of Michigan Health System, 24 Frank Lloyd Wright Drive, Lobby A, P.O. Box 391, Ann Arbor, MI 48106, USA; [c] The Hip, James M. Benson Sports Rehabilitation Center, Belaire Building, Ground Floor, 525 East 71st Street, New York, NY 10021, USA; [d] Sports Medicine and Shoulder Surgery, Domino's Farms – MedSport, University of Michigan Health System, 24 Frank Lloyd Wright Drive, Lobby A, P.O. Box 391, Ann Arbor, MI 48106, USA
* Corresponding author.
E-mail address: abedi@med.umich.edu

Clin Sports Med 35 (2016) 637–654
http://dx.doi.org/10.1016/j.csm.2016.05.008
0278-5919/16/$ – see front matter © 2016 Elsevier Inc. All rights reserved.

presentations commonly occur as a combination of the 2 pathomorphologies (combined-type lesion). Although the concept of FAI was first described by Smith-Peterson in 1936,[1] it was Ganz and colleagues[2] who pioneered much of the modern modalities used for the diagnosis and treatment of the disorder, elucidating the pathophysiology that creates abnormal loading mechanics and results in secondary degenerative changes within the hip joint.[3,4]

Mechanical impingement at the terminal range of hip motion resultant from this pathology often causes tearing or detachment of the acetabular labrum from the articular cartilage.[5] During dynamic cyclic hip motion, repetitive impaction and abnormal regional loading of the femoral head-neck junction against the acetabular rim may cause microtrauma and chondral delamination.[3,6–10] Localization of these injuries reflect the topography of the deformity, and are typically at the anterosuperior region of the acetabular rim with concomitant disruption at the adjacent transition zone of the articular cartilage. Early diagnosis and management of these injuries are critical, as their severity often correlates with the severity of the pathomorphology and the time between symptom onset and treatment.[11–15] FAI may be particularly disabling to the high-demand athlete with significant cutting and pivoting requirements, therefore a clear understanding of the etiology, diagnosis, management, and outcomes is essential for clinicians to optimally help patients to return to play.[16]

FEMOROACETABULAR IMPINGEMENT IN ATHLETES
Etiology

A significant number of athletes present with hip pain and functional disability due to FAI.[17–19] Symptomatic hip pain related to FAI is commonly diagnosed with athletic activities that may require end ranges of motion. Examples include cutting motions and repeated changes of direction as seen in soccer, increased hip flexion/abduction/internal rotation as seen in ice hockey, and supraphysiological ranges of motion as seen in dance.[20] These athletes often push their hips to extreme ranges of motion, particularly with internal rotation. The full spectrum of competition levels is represented, from recreational weekend warriors to elite professional athletes.[21,22] In addition, symptomatic FAI has been demonstrated to be more common in certain types of athletes as compared with the general population.[23–26]

Increased prevalence of femoroacetabular impingement in athletes

Gerhardt and colleagues[25] showed that the prevalence of FAI among 95 elite male and female soccer players was high, with 70% cam-type and 50% pincer-type lesions observed on radiographs. In a comparative study evaluating 22 asymptomatic male semiprofessional and 22 amateur male soccer players (median age: 23.3; range: 18–30 years), Lahner and colleagues[27] demonstrated that the mean kicking leg alpha angle in the semiprofessional group ($57.3 \pm 8.2°$) was significantly higher as compared with the amateur group ($51.7 \pm 4.8°$, $P = .008$). In a sample of 123 hips with a history of hip or groin pain obtained from athletes at the National Football League Combine, Nepple and colleagues[28] determined that 94.3% demonstrated radiographic evidence for FAI (cam-type: 98%; pincer-type: 22.8%; combined-type: 61.8%). Larson and colleagues[19] corroborated these findings with another study evaluating a mixed cohort of 238 symptomatic and asymptomatic hips from the National Football League Combine, noting that 87% exhibited at least one radiographic sign consistent with FAI and determining that increasing alpha angle was an independent predictor for the development of groin pain.

Mariconda and colleagues[29] examined radiographs from 24 experienced capoeira players (a Brazilian martial art that requires extreme movements of the hip to perform jumps and kicks) and found that 91.7% hips had signs for cam-type lesions and 37.5% had signs for pincer-type lesions, with a subsequent 33.3% of hips demonstrating combined-type FAI. Similar findings are also present in track and field athletes, as Lahner and colleagues[30] demonstrated that 22 elite athletes (52.2 ± 7.29°) had significantly greater alpha angles when compared with controls (48.1 ± 5.45°, $P = .004$). In addition, the prevalence of symptomatic FAI is not limited to sports primarily focused on the lower extremities. Klingenstein and colleagues[31] treated 34 high-level overhead athletes (baseball and lacrosse players; mean age: 21.4 years; range, 16–35 years) presenting with symptomatic FAI.

Development of femoroacetabular impingement during skeletal maturity

Increasing levels of high physical activity in adolescents has been postulated as a contributing factor in developing FAI.[26,32,33] Agricola and colleagues[26] demonstrated in 89 elite pre-professional soccer players and 92 controls (age range: 12–19 years) that cam-type lesions on radiographs were identified significantly more often in soccer players as compared with their nonathletic peer controls (elite: 13%; controls: 0%, $P<.03$). The investigators found cam-type lesions in athletes as young as 13 years.[26] Agricola and colleagues[34] subsequently reported on the radiographs of 63 pre-professional soccer players (mean age: 14.43 years; range: 12–19 years) at baseline and at a mean 2.4-year subsequent follow-up. The prevalence of a head-neck prominence significantly increased from 2.1% to 17.7% ($P = .002$) in hips with an open growth plate at baseline, with no significant increase in the prevalence or size of the cam-lesion following growth plate closure.[34] The alpha angle was also significantly increased from 59.4° at baseline to 61.3° at follow-up ($P = .018$). The investigators concluded that cam-type lesions may gradually develop during the period of skeletal immaturity and could potentially be ameliorated through modification of athletic activity during this time.[34]

Philippon and colleagues[35] analyzed 61 asymptomatic youth ice hockey players (age range: 10–18 years) along with 27 youth control skiers (age range: 10–18 years) and found that the ice hockey players had significantly higher alpha angles as compared with controls (75% vs 42% with an alpha angle >55°, $P<.006$). Similar findings have been demonstrated in youth ice hockey players, as Siebenrock and colleagues[21] evaluated a group of 77 elite athletes (mean age: 16.5 years; range: 9–36 years) and found that alpha angles were increased in patients with closed growth plates (58°) as compared with patients with open growth plates (49°: $P<.001$). This suggests that elite-level ice hockey participation during skeletal development may be associated with an increased risk for developing cam-type lesions.

The currently available evidence suggests that development of FAI for the young athlete potentially starts at an early age during skeletal maturity. Nepple and colleagues[36] performed a systematic review analyzing the development of FAI in association with sporting activity in adolescence and demonstrated that boys participating in high-level impact sports have an increased risk of cam-lesion presentation. High-level male athletes were 1.9 to 8.0 times more likely to develop a cam-lesion, with a 41% cam-lesion prevalence as compared with 17% in controls. The biomechanical stresses that the femoroacetabular joint experiences during repetitive physical activity may result in focal patterns of abnormal force on the growth plate and surrounding bone. The highly dynamic and cyclic nature of increased impact activity resulting from certain sports may generate higher mechanical joint loading with subsequent growth stimulus. These abnormal mechanical loads are produced at the extreme ranges of hip motion and therefore may be applied at areas of the joint that are relatively naïve to these types of loads. The current trend of early sports specialization may compound this effect for an even greater degree of deformity development, due to exceeding volume or intensity workload thresholds.

Demographics

Nawabi and colleagues[20] recently performed a retrospective review of 622 athletes (288 high-level, 334 recreational) who underwent hip arthroscopy for FAI in an attempt to determine demographic differences in age, gender, and the need for bilateral surgery for high-level athletes as compared with recreational athletes. The investigators determined that high-level athletes were associated with younger age (mean age: 20.2 vs 33.0 years; odds ratio: 0.69; $P<.001$) and male gender (61.5% vs 53.6%; odds ratio: 1.75; $P = .03$). The investigators also found that high-level athletes received bilateral surgery more frequently (28.4% vs 15.9%); however, the significance of this relationship was determined to be confounded by age. High-level male athletes undergoing surgery most commonly participated in ice hockey followed by football, as compared with high-level female athletes who most frequently participated in soccer followed by dance. Cutting sport athletes (soccer, basketball, lacrosse, and field hockey) represented the largest group of patients by sports category, followed by athletes involved in impingement sports (ice hockey, crew/rowing, baseball catcher, water polo, equestrian polo, and breaststroke swimmer). Cutting athletes underwent surgical management at a significantly younger age (19.2 years) as compared with flexibility athletes (dance, gymnastics, yoga, cheer, figure skating, and martial arts) (20.9 years; $P = .03$), contact athletes (football, rugby, and wrestling) (mean age: 21.3 years; $P = .005$), and impingement athletes (mean age: 21.3 years; $P<.001$). Athletes performing flexibility sports underwent ligamentum teres debridement significantly more frequently as compared with impingement sports ($P = .004$) and asymmetric sports (baseball, softball, tennis, golf, volleyball, and field events) ($P = .03$).

These findings highlight that there may be important differences between athletes of different sports with corresponding implications for management and correction of deformity. In addition to age-related factors, the unique biomechanical demands on the hip applied by different categories of sport may significantly influence the development of symptomatic FAI in varying athletes. For example, the flexibility athletes are a unique group in that rehabilitation philosophy is different compared with the cutting athlete. Rehabilitation focus is on mobility in the more standard FAI patient, such as the cutting athlete, whereas undercovered patients with FAI, such as flexibility athletes, have a focus on neuromuscular stability. The category of sport may be predictive of a particular pattern of intra-articular damage or compensatory pathology. Krych and colleagues[37] performed a retrospective review to analyze 22 mixed-sport athletes presenting with posterior acetabular rim fractures with subsequent posterior instability and found that 81.8% had alpha angles greater than 45° and 77.3% had associated ligamentum teres avulsion, suggesting an association between these pathologies. Nawabi and colleagues[20] also demonstrated significantly more frequent findings of ligament teres pathology, but these were more common in flexibility athletes. Awareness of varying demographics among different groups of athletes are important to identify the individual needs of patients when considering preventive, nonoperative, or surgical management options.

SURGICAL TREATMENT OPTIONS
Surgical Hip Dislocation

Preservation of the native intra-articular hip environment and prevention of early-onset arthritis are the most important goals in hip preservation surgery. Hip surgery aims to address intra-articular damage caused by FAI, particularly labral tears and articular cartilage lesions.[38] The specific surgical approach must be individualized for each patient to adequately address the pattern and extent of intra-articular pathology. The classic open procedure to address symptomatic FAI is the surgical hip dislocation as described by Ganz and colleagues[2]; however, other techniques include the Smith-Peterson approach, and the Heurter anterior arthrotomy.[39,40]

The surgical hip dislocation allows for complete visualization of the acetabular rim and femoral head-neck junction by using a trochanteric slide osteotomy and using the short external rotator muscles to preserve femoral head blood supply. Naal and colleagues[41] evaluated 22 professional male athletes (mean age: 19.7 ± 2.2 years) following surgical dislocation and found that 96% continued to compete professionally at an average of 45.1 months, with 19 patients participating at their previous level. Novais and colleagues[42] analyzed a group of 29 young athletes with symptomatic FAI (mean age: 17 years; range 12.7–20.7 years) who were managed with surgical hip dislocation with a mean follow-up of 1.8 years. These investigators concluded that 80% of these patients either improved their athletic activity level or maintained it at the maximum possible level, in addition to significantly improved pain scores following surgical dislocation.[42] Bizzini and colleagues[43] evaluated 5 young professional ice hockey players (mean age: 21.4 years) who underwent surgical decompression of the hip with a mean follow-up of 2.7 years and found that hip rotation range of motion was regained by 10.3 weeks, hip strength values reach preoperative levels by a mean of 7.8 months, return to unrestricted team practice was achieved by a mean of 6.7 months, and participation in competitive games occurred after a mean of 9.6 months. However, although 3 athletes were able to return to preoperative international level of competition, 2 patients were able to return only as minor league players.[43]

Although surgical dislocation has been shown to achieve extensive access to the native hip for surgical management of FAI, significant complications of the procedure are reported in approximately 6%.[44] These include trochanteric bursitis secondary to prominent hardware (26%), trochanteric nonunion (3%–20%), heterotopic ossification (3%), and uncommonly femoral head osteonecrosis, and persistent weakness of the hip abductors.[44–46]

Hip Arthroscopy

Rapid advances in hip arthroscopy to address symptomatic FAI has allowed for extensive visualization and management of joint pathology. The primary techniques include femoral osteochondroplasty to address the cam-lesion and acetabular rim-resection to address the pincer-lesion. Labral injury may necessitate refixation, debridement, or reconstruction depending on the tissue quality at the time of surgery. In addition, articular cartilage damage due to abnormal joint surface forces may be addressed with microfracture techniques. Botser and colleagues[47] showed in a systematic review that hip arthroscopy provides improved return to play rates and decreased complication rates for professional athletes compared with open surgical hip dislocation, potentially due to the minimally invasive nature of the operation. There have been 2 previous systematic reviews on the rate of return to play following surgery for FAI that demonstrate favorable outcomes.[48,49]

Importance of early diagnosis and management

Return to play outcomes following hip arthroscopy in the current literature have demonstrated positive results. Philippon and colleagues[50] analyzed 28 elite National Hockey League athletes (mean age: 27 years; range: 18–37) and found that all athletes were able to initially return to competitive play, participating in an average of 94 professional games postoperatively. However, there was a significant variability in sustained return to play at an elite level, as the number of games played ranged from 3 to 252. The investigators described a negative correlation between age and number of games played postoperatively ($R = -0.48$; $P = .009$). A positive correlation between time to surgery and time to return to play was also present ($r = 0.582$; $P = .001$), with athletes undergoing hip arthroscopy within 1 year of injury returning to play at an average of 3 months as opposed to athletes undergoing surgery beyond 1 year of injury, returning to play at an average of 4.1 months. In an earlier study that analyzed 45 mixed-sport professional athletes, Philippon and colleagues[51] also found that 42 (93%) patients were able to return to professional competition at an average of 1.6 years (range: 6 months–5.5 years).

Similar findings are present in a study by Sansone and colleagues[52] analyzing 85 top-level athletes (mean age: 25 ± 5 years), which used the Hip Sports Activity Scale (HSAS) to determine the level of competition to which the athlete returned postoperatively. Athletes receiving treatment within 12 months of the onset of symptoms not only had a significantly higher rate of return to play (87% vs 61%, $P<.05$), but also returned to their previous competition level at a significantly higher rate as compared with athletes surgically managed beyond 12 months of symptom duration (74% vs 64%, $P<.05$). This literature suggests that early detection and appropriate management of the athlete with symptomatic FAI is a crucial factor in return to play. Progressive tissue damage and inferior outcomes may be perpetuated with delayed diagnosis, particularly in the context of continued high-intensity activity at the professional level.

Professional and nonprofessional athletes

Although much of the existing literature focuses on professional athletes, several investigators also have evaluated outcomes in the nonprofessional athlete undergoing hip arthroscopy. Brunner and colleagues[53] analyzed 45 recreational athletes (mean age: 41 years; range: 17–66 years) and found that only 4 of these patients were participating at their normal level at the time of initial presentation, with the remaining patients performing either below their normal level (n = 13) or had stopped participating in sports altogether (n = 28). Thirty-one (68.9%) were able to return to their previous level of activity at a mean follow-up of 2.4 years postoperatively (range: 2–3.2 years). Using the sports frequency scale (grade 0: no sports activity; grade 1: moderate level of activity, <1 h/wk; grade 2: normal level of activity, 1–5 h/wk; grade 3: high level of activity, >5 h/wk; grade 4: professional level of activity, elite athlete), there was a significant increase in activity level at final follow-up as compared with preoperative baseline (0.78 vs 1.84 $P<.001$).

Nho and colleagues[54] analyzed a mixed group of 47 high-level athletes (27.7% varsity high school, 53.2% college, and 19.1% professional; mean age: 22.8 ± 6.2 years) with a minimum follow-up of 1 year. Of the 33 athletes who were available for follow-up, 26 (79%) were able to return to play at a mean of 9.4 ± 4.7 months (range: 4–26 months) postoperatively with 24 of those athletes (92.3%) returning to the same level of competition. These 24 athletes continued participating in competition at 2 years, but the level of competition at this point was not reported. The rate of return was 90% (9 of 10) in high school athletes, 59% (10 of 17) in collegiate athletes, and 83% (5 of 6) in professional athletes. Of the 7 athletes who were unable to return to play, 5 were due to persistent hip pain. Byrd and Jones[55] performed an analysis of 200 athletic patients (28.6 years; range, 11–60 years), including 23 professional, 56 intercollegiate, 24 high school, and 97 recreational athletes. A total of 181 athletes

(90%) returned to their previous level of competition, with 95% returning at the professional level and 85% at the collegiate level and an average follow-up of 19 months (range: 12–60 months).

Malviya and colleagues[56] demonstrated similar findings in a comparative analysis of 40 professional and 40 recreational athletes (mean age: 35.7 years; range: 14–59 years) with a mean follow-up of 1.4 years (range: 1–1.8 years). The average return to sport duration was 5.4 months (range: 3–10 months) for all athletes, but professional athletes required significantly less time (mean: 4.2 months) as compared with recreational athletes (mean: 6.8 months, $P = .03$). All athletes followed the same rehabilitation protocol, so the differential motivational or fitness aspects between professional and recreational athletes may explain this finding. Both professional and recreational groups demonstrated high rates of return to play at 6 months (78% and 65%, respectively) and 1 year (82% and 73%, respectively) without significant differences. There was a 2.6-fold improvement in the training time after surgery and a 3.2-fold increase in the time in competition 1 year after surgery. Although professional and nonprofessional athletes both demonstrated good outcomes, the literature suggests that professional athletes may exhibit superior rate of return to play and faster return to play time. Professional athletes also returned to their previous level of activity at a higher rate. A potential explanation for this observation could be that professional athletes hold significantly greater socioeconomic investment in their sport and therefore possess elevated motivation for return to play. This information can be useful in setting appropriate expectations for athletes of different competition levels.

Adolescent athletes

As the age of athletes competing in sustained high-level activity continues to become younger, the incidence of hip pathology in this population has progressively risen and the use of hip arthroscopy for their management has become increasingly common.[57] However, the benefits of surgery must be balanced with the potential complications of joint incongruity and early osteoarthritis, avascular necrosis, slipped capital femoral epiphysis, and physeal arrest resulting from operating on an athlete with open growth plates.[58] Philippon and colleagues[59] retrospectively evaluated 16 adolescent athletes (mean age: 15 years, range: 11–16 years) and found significant improvements in the modified Harris Hip Scale (mHHS), the Hip Outcome Score Activities of Daily Living (HOS ADL) and Sport Specific subscale (HOS SS), and satisfaction scores ($P<.05$ for all) at an average follow-up of 1.36 years (range, 1–2 years); however, no return to play results were reported. No cases of osteonecrosis or growth abnormalities were reported following surgery. Tran and colleagues[60] reported on 34 adolescent athletes (41 hips; mean age: 15.7 years; range: 11–18 years) with open proximal femoral growth plates and found that 32 athletes (94.1%) were able to return to play at an average follow-up of 14 months (range: 1–2 years). Twenty-five athletes (78.1%) returned to their previous level of competition, 4 (12.5%) returned at a lower level, and 3 (8.8%) were unable to return to sport. Overall, 30 (88.2%) of the 34 athletes were satisfied and 31 (91.2%) would undergo surgery again. The investigators reported no incidences of avascular necrosis, physeal growth plate arrest, acute slipped capital femoral epiphysis, or other significant complications. In both studies, limited femoral osteochondroplasties were performed for patients with open physeal plates.

These findings are mirrored in an analysis by Fabricant and colleagues[61] observing 21 adolescent athletes (27 hips; mean age 17.6 ± 1.6 years), which found significant improvements in the mHHS (66–88, $P<.001$), HOS ADL (77–92, $P<.0001$), and HOS SS (49–82, $P=.001$). In contrast to the previous studies, all patients in this cohort were skeletally mature and received complete femoral osteochondroplasty procedures.

Although the investigators do not report specific return to play rates, all athletes reported either "Normal" (37.0%) or "Nearly Normal" (63.0%) on a self-reported hip outcome score in relation to sport function at follow-up as compared with baseline. A recent systematic review by de Sa and colleagues[62] demonstrated that hip arthroscopy in skeletally immature patients appear to be safe and efficacious in treating symptomatic FAI. Hip arthroscopy for adolescent athletes appears to produce generally positive short-term results with high rates of return to play and satisfaction. The operation has been considered to be safe, as complications stemming from surgery on an open proximal femoral physis have not been reported in the current literature. Long-term prospective research is required to determine if these benefits are maintained and whether hip arthroscopy alters the progression toward early hip osteoarthritis for these young athletes.

Chondral damage, osteoarthritis, and microfracture in athletes

Articular cartilage damage commonly occurs with the abnormal mechanical loads induced onto the joint by symptomatic FAI. Transition zone shear injuries with adjacent cartilage damage is typically caused during repetitive entry of cam-lesions into the joint, subsequently resulting in chondral delamination.[63] Pincer-lesions commonly result in posteroinferior articular contrecoup damage due to the levering effect of the acetabular overcoverage, creating abnormal sheer forces on posterior chondral surfaces.[38] These chondral injuries may result in significant pain and functional deficit in the active athlete. Singh and O'Donnell[64] analyzed 24 professional Australian Football League players (mean age: 22 years, range: 16–29 years) and found that the only athlete who was unable to return to play demonstrated greater than 40% chondral loss on intraoperative examination, whereas the 23 (96%) other athletes had substantially less cartilage damage and were able to return to their previous level of professional play at a mean follow-up of 22 months (range: 6–60 months).

Microfracture at the time of hip arthroscopy has been developed to manage these focal chondral injuries.[65] To evaluate the utility of hip arthroscopy in the management of chondral lesions in elite athletes, McDonald and colleagues[66] recently performed a comparative study between 39 male hips that underwent microfracture for discrete Outerbridge grade IV chondral lesions and 94 male control hips without microfracture. The 2 groups did not significantly differ in terms of return to play, as 30 athletes (77%) undergoing microfracture were able to return to competition at some point as compared with 79 control athletes (84%). Interestingly, 22 athletes (70%) undergoing microfracture continued professional play an average of 3 seasons postoperatively (range: 1–11 seasons), whereas only 43 control athletes (54%) continued professional play an average of 2.8 seasons (range: 1–11 seasons); however, there was no statistically significant difference detected. In the cohort of 200 mixed-level athletes reported by Byrd and colleagues,[55] 88% had Outerbridge grade III or grade IV articular damage. Forty-nine of those athletes underwent microfracture surgery with a resultant 92% return to play rate postoperatively, similar to athletes undergoing hip arthroscopy without the additional microfracture procedure.

Although the natural history of these chondral lesions is unclear, the current literature suggests that these injuries may continue to progress in severity and ultimately result in early-onset hip osteoarthritis if left unmanaged.[67] Byrd and Jones[68] followed 15 athletes (mean age: 31.7 years; range: 14–70 years) who underwent hip arthroscopy and analyzed their return to play at minimum follow-up of 10 years. Although 13 (87%) athletes were initially able to return to play, 5 of these patients were eventually deemed failures. The investigators found that all 5 of these athletes presented with arthritis at the time of surgery, all of whom progressed to total hip arthroplasty at an average of 73 months (range: 4–119 months) and demonstrated significantly inferior outcomes (P<.006). Additionally, the retrospective analysis of 45 mixed-sport professional athletes reviewed earlier by Philippon and colleagues[51] concluded that the presence of diffuse osteoarthritis was a predictor for worse postoperative outcomes, as all 5 patients with this finding were unable to ultimately return to play.

When management is initiated in the athlete before radiographic signs of significant osteoarthritis, athletes are generally able to return to competition. For microfracture to be effective, it is important that the athlete commit to follow a consistent postoperative and rehabilitation protocol.[65] Taken together, athletes undergoing additional microfracture procedures for focal chondral defects secondary to FAI exhibit high rates of return to play, with competition-level durability similar to other athletes without chondral defects. However, athletes receiving microfracture must have a high level of commitment to the rehabilitation process if they are to receive a good outcome. Platelet-rich plasma is an evolving technique as a conjunction to hip arthroscopy in the setting of articular damage and early osteoarthritis. Although some studies have demonstrated some improved tissue healing, the body of literature is lacking and needs and higher levels of evidence are required to infer any clinical utility for athletes.[69]

Labral reconstruction in athletes

Disruption of the longitudinal fibers may functionally cripple the labrum and provide minimal viable tissue to primarily repair, necessitating a reconstruction technique with tissue grafting.[70] Clinical and functional outcomes have demonstrated positive results in the general population; however, specific literature focusing on athletes is sparse.[71] The restoration of a competent labrum is especially important in the athletic population, as the return of physiologic hip biomechanics is critical to achieve the mobility necessary to these patients. Boykin and colleagues[72] performed a retrospective review of 21 elite athletes (23 hips; mean age: 28.0 years; range: 19–41 years) who underwent hip arthroscopy for labral reconstruction with iliotibial band graft with an average follow-up of 41.4 months (range: 20–74 months). The investigators determined that the athletes achieved a high rate of return to play of 18 athletes (85.7%), 17 (81%) of whom returned to a similar level of competition. The investigators also found significant improvements in the mHHS (67–84, P = .026) and HOS SS (56–77, P = .009). However, 2 patients eventually progressed to arthroplasty.[72]

In a systematic review evaluating outcomes following labral reconstruction, Ayeni and colleagues[71] concluded that the ideal candidates for the technique were young, active patients with more than 2 mm of joint space preservation. Philippon and colleagues[70] found that patient age was an independent predictor for patient satisfaction for a general population undergoing labral reconstruction with iliotibial band. The average age of the 9% progressing to total hip arthroplasty in this cohort was significantly older as compared with those who did not require replacement (49 years vs 36 years, P = .027). The 2 athletes who progressed to arthroplasty in the study by Boykin and colleagues[71] were older (37 and 31 years) compared with the other patients and exhibited evidence of osteoarthritis and less than 2 mm joint space preservation on radiographs. Both of these factors have been shown to be independent predictors of hip arthroscopy failure. The available evidence is limited, but labral reconstruction appears to provide improved short-term outcomes and good return to play rates in the younger athletic population that does not have evidence of osteoarthritis. Longer-term prospective studies will be required to evaluate the durability of these grafts to preserve high-level functioning and to mitigate early-onset osteoarthritis.

Table 1
Hip arthroscopy rehabilitation: labral repair with or without femoroacetabular impingement component

Postoperative Time Period	Rehabilitation Activities and Progressions
Weeks 0–2	• Focus on decreasing soft tissue swelling and restoring gliding of adjacent tissues • Stationary bicycle for 20 min/d (up to twice a day) • ROM progression – Stool rotations (AAROM Hip IR), pelvic tilts, supine hip log rolling, limit external rotation to <20° (**Fig. 1**) • Hip isometrics (no flexion): prone leg curls, prone abdominal/gluteal/quad-hamstring/dorsiflexion isometric holds, quadruped hand heel rocks with stable core, supine bridges • Neuromuscular electrical stimulation to quadriceps with short arc quadriceps if indicated or appropriate • Sustained stretching for psoas with cryotherapy (2 pillows under hips) • Gait training every session to prevent the development of poor motion
Weeks 2–4	• Progress weight bearing: wean off crutches at weeks 3–4 • Progress hip ROM as tolerated: bent knee fall outs (week 4), stool rotations for ER (weeks 3–4), hip hiking (week 4) • Gluteal/piriformis stretching • Progress core and hip strengthening (avoid hip flexor tendonitis): bilateral cable column rotations (weeks 3–4) (**Fig. 2**), isotonic exercises (no flexion), clam shells→isometric side lying hip abduction (**Fig. 3**) • Step ups and downs starting with 4″ box building to 8″ box • Begin proprioception/balance training: balance boards, single leg stance (**Fig. 4**) • Aquatic therapy in low end of water
Weeks 4–8	• Progress strengthening: introduce hip flexion prone isometrics to AAROM, multi-hip machine (open and closed chain), leg press (bilateral →unilateral), single leg wall push, windmills, lawn mowers, resistive hip hikes (begin with doing all exercises as the stance leg first to ensure muscular strength, endurance, and neuromuscular control before the moving leg) (**Fig. 5**) • Progress core strengthening: prone/side planks • Progress proprioception/balance: standing rotations with rocker bottom boards • Treadmill side-stepping (week 6) • Elliptical (weeks 4–6) • Hip flexor, gluteus/piriformis, and IT band stretching: seated eccentric hip flexor stretch (**Fig. 6**) • 3-Point step with theraband progressing to side-stepping with theraband (**Fig. 7**)
Weeks 8–12	• Progressive hip ROM • Progressive extremity and core strengthening using challenging surfaces or perturbations • Endurance activities around the hip • Dynamic balance activities
Weeks 12–16	• Progressive extremity and core strengthening • Plyometrics: begin with in-place double leg progressing to single leg jumps, hops and bounds being sure to monitor sets, foot contacts, and rest between sets • Begin treadmill or field running program • Sport-specific agility drills • Return to supervised modified weight room program • Begin developing a time-based plan for return to activity and sport

Abbreviations: AAROM, active assistive range of motion; ER, external rotation; IR, internal rotation; IT, iliotibial; ROM, range of motion.

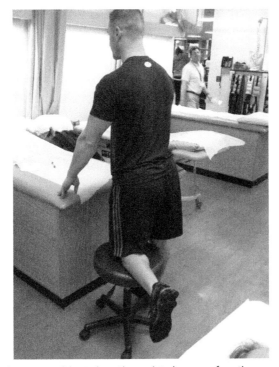

Fig. 1. Stool rotations to participate in active assisted range of motion exercises, particularly hip internal/external rotation.

REHABILITATION

Postoperative rehabilitation protocols should include activities that accurately evaluate an athlete's physical status and determine appropriate progressions for safe return to play. **Table 1** demonstrates our preferred progression of rehabilitation with specific activity examples.

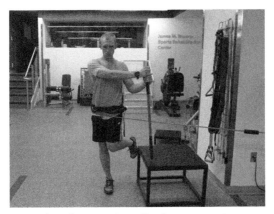

Fig. 2. Cable column rotations for core strengthening progression.

A

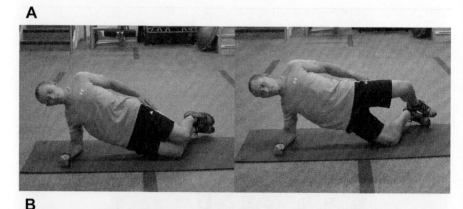

B

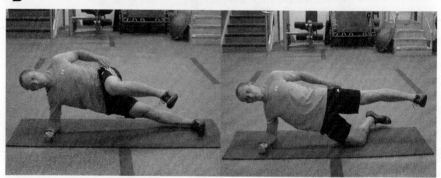

Fig. 3. (*A*) Clam shell exercise for hip external rotation and abduction. (*B*) Progression to isometric side-lying hip abduction.

SUMMARY

Intra-articular pathology leading to symptomatic hip pain results in significant morbidity and functional deficits in the young athlete. Symptomatic FAI is the most common cause of prearthritic hip pain in the nondysplastic hip. If nonoperative

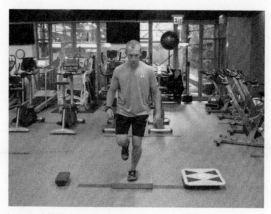

Fig. 4. Proprioception and balance training using a variety of devices.

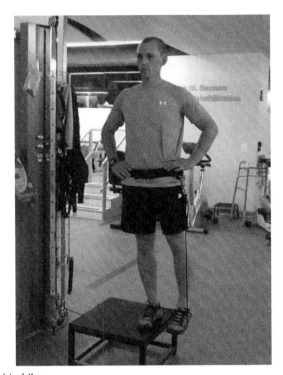

Fig. 5. Resistive hip hikes.

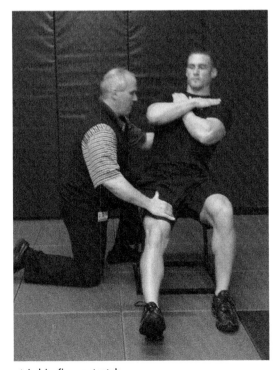

Fig. 6. Seated eccentric hip flexor stretch.

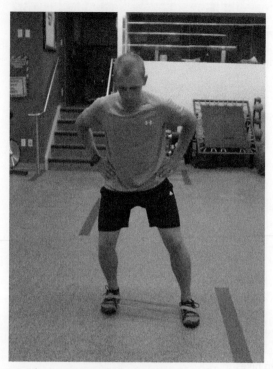

Fig. 7. Progressing to side-stepping with theraband.

treatment fails to adequately alleviate symptoms or sufficiently restore function in the athlete, hip arthroscopy can lead to improved pain, improved range of motion, and high rates of return to play with proper postoperative rehabilitation. The rate of return to previous level of competition is also high with accurate diagnosis and well-executed correction of deformity. Important considerations include the ability to achieve the diagnosis in a timely manner and to exercise caution in older athletes with presence of preexisting osteoarthritis or diminished joint space. Expectations should be managed in these patients, as the literature demonstrates suboptimal outcomes in these populations. Higher quality of evidence with long-term prospective studies are required to determine the effectiveness of this technique to durably maintain athletes in athletic activity and alter the natural history of disease progression.

REFERENCES

1. Smith-Petersen MN. The classic: treatment of malum coxae senilis, old slipped upper femoral epiphysis, intrapelvic protrusion of the acetabulum, and coxa plana by means of acetabuloplasty. 1936. Clin Orthop Relat Res 2009;467(3): 608–15.
2. Ganz R, Leunig M, Leunig-Ganz K, et al. The etiology of osteoarthritis of the hip: an integrated mechanical concept. Clin Orthop Relat Res 2008;466(2):264–72.
3. Ganz R, Parvizi J, Beck M, et al. Femoroacetabular impingement: a cause for osteoarthritis of the hip. Clin Orthop Relat Res 2003;417:112–20.
4. Ganz R, Gill TJ, Gautier E, et al. Surgical dislocation of the adult hip: a technique with full access to the femoral head and acetabulum without the risk of avascular necrosis. J Bone Joint Surg Br 2001;83(8):1119–24.

5. Wenger DE, Kendell KR, Miner MR, et al. Acetabular labral tears rarely occur in the absence of bony abnormalities. Clin Orthop Relat Res 2004;426:145–50.
6. Khanduja V, Villar RN. Arthroscopic surgery of the hip: current concepts and recent advances. J Bone Joint Surg Br 2006;88(12):1557–66.
7. Crawford JR, Villar RN. Current concepts in the management of femoroacetabular impingement. J Bone Joint Surg Br 2005;87(11):1459–62.
8. Bedi A, Chen N, Robertson W, et al. The management of labral tears and femoroacetabular impingement of the hip in the young, active patient. Arthroscopy 2008;24(10):1135–45.
9. Anderson LA, Peters CL, Park BB, et al. Acetabular cartilage delamination in femoroacetabular impingement. J Bone Joint Surg Am 2009;91(2):305–13.
10. Allen D, Beaulé PE, Ramadan O, et al. Prevalence of associated deformities and hip pain in patients with cam-type femoroacetabular impingement. J Bone Joint Surg Br 2009;91(5):589–94.
11. Nepple JJ, Zebala LP, Clohisy JC. Labral disease associated with femoroacetabular impingement: do we need to correct the structural deformity? J Arthroplasty 2009;24(6 Suppl):114–9.
12. Kelly BT, Weiland DE, Schenker ML, et al. Arthroscopic labral repair in the hip: surgical technique and review of the literature. Arthroscopy 2005;21(12): 1496–504.
13. Johnston TL, Schenker ML, Briggs KK, et al. Relationship between offset angle alpha and hip chondral injury in femoroacetabular impingement. Arthroscopy 2008;24(6):669–75.
14. Dolan MM, Heyworth BE, Bedi A, et al. CT reveals a high incidence of osseous abnormalities in hips with labral tears. Clin Orthop Relat Res 2011;469(3):831–8.
15. Burnett RSJ, Rocca GJD, Prather H, et al. Clinical presentation of patients with tears of the acetabular labrum. J Bone Joint Surg Am 2006;88(7):1448–57.
16. Bennell K, Hunter DJ, Vicenzino B. Long-term effects of sport: preventing and managing OA in the athlete. Nat Rev Rheumatol 2012;8(12):747–52.
17. Yuan BJ, Bartelt RB, Levy BA, et al. Decreased range of motion is associated with structural hip deformity in asymptomatic adolescent athletes. Am J Sports Med 2013;41(7):1519–25.
18. Weir A, de Vos RJ, Moen M, et al. Prevalence of radiological signs of femoroacetabular impingement in patients presenting with long-standing adductor-related groin pain. Br J Sports Med 2011;45(1):6–9.
19. Larson CM, Sikka RS, Sardelli MC, et al. Increasing alpha angle is predictive of athletic-related "hip" and "groin" pain in collegiate National Football League prospects. Arthroscopy 2013;29(3):405–10.
20. Nawabi DH, Bedi A, Tibor LM, et al. The demographic characteristics of high-level and recreational athletes undergoing hip arthroscopy for femoroacetabular impingement: a sports-specific analysis. Arthroscopy 2014;30(3):398–405.
21. Siebenrock KA, Kaschka I, Frauchiger L, et al. Prevalence of cam-type deformity and hip pain in elite ice hockey players before and after the end of growth. Am J Sports Med 2013;41(10):2308–13.
22. Hammoud S, Bedi A, Magennis E, et al. High incidence of athletic pubalgia symptoms in professional athletes with symptomatic femoroacetabular impingement. Arthroscopy 2012;28(10):1388–95.
23. Silvis ML, Mosher TJ, Smetana BS, et al. High prevalence of pelvic and hip magnetic resonance imaging findings in Asymptomatic Collegiate and Professional Hockey Players. Am J Sports Med 2011;39(4):715–21.

24. Kapron AL, Anderson AE, Aoki SK, et al. Radiographic prevalence of femoroacetabular impingement in collegiate football players: AAOS Exhibit Selection. J Bone Joint Surg Am 2011;93(19). e111(1–10).
25. Gerhardt MB, Romero AA, Silvers HJ, et al. The prevalence of radiographic hip abnormalities in elite soccer players. Am J Sports Med 2012;40(3):584–8.
26. Agricola R, Bessems JHJM, Ginai AZ, et al. The development of cam-type deformity in adolescent and young male soccer players. Am J Sports Med 2012;40(5): 1099–106.
27. Lahner M, Walter PA, von Schulze Pellengahr C, et al. Comparative study of the femoroacetabular impingement (FAI) prevalence in male semiprofessional and amateur soccer players. Arch Orthop Trauma Surg 2014;134(8):1135–41.
28. Nepple JJ, Brophy RH, Matava MJ, et al. Radiographic findings of femoroacetabular impingement in National Football League Combine athletes undergoing radiographs for previous hip or groin pain. Arthroscopy 2012;28(10):1396–403.
29. Mariconda M, Cozzolino A, Di Pietto F, et al. Radiographic findings of femoroacetabular impingement in capoeira players. Knee Surg Sports Traumatol Arthrosc 2014;22(4):874–81.
30. Lahner M, Bader S, Walter PA, et al. Prevalence of femoro-acetabular impingement in international competitive track and field athletes. Int Orthop 2014; 38(12):2571–6.
31. Klingenstein GG, Martin R, Kivlan B, et al. Hip injuries in the overhead athlete. Clin Orthop Relat Res 2012;470(6):1579–85.
32. Bedi A, Lynch EB, Sibilsky Enselman ER, et al. Elevation in circulating biomarkers of cartilage damage and inflammation in athletes with femoroacetabular impingement. Am J Sports Med 2013;41(11):2585–90.
33. Philippon MJ, Stubbs AJ, Schenker ML, et al. Arthroscopic management of femoroacetabular impingement: osteoplasty technique and literature review. Am J Sports Med 2007;35(9):1571–80.
34. Agricola R, Heijboer MP, Ginai AZ, et al. A cam deformity is gradually acquired during skeletal maturation in adolescent and young male soccer players: a prospective study with minimum 2-year follow-up. Am J Sports Med 2014;42(4): 798–806.
35. Philippon MJ, Ho CP, Briggs KK, et al. Prevalence of increased alpha angles as a measure of cam-type femoroacetabular impingement in youth ice hockey players. Am J Sports Med 2013;41(6):1357–62.
36. Nepple JJ, Vigdorchik JM, Clohisy JC. What is the association between sports participation and the development of proximal femoral cam deformity? A systematic review and meta-analysis. Am J Sports Med 2015;43(11):2833–40.
37. Krych AJ, Thompson M, Larson CM, et al. Is posterior hip instability associated with cam and pincer deformity? Clin Orthop Relat Res 2012;470(12):3390–7.
38. Bedi A, Dolan M, Leunig M, et al. Static and dynamic mechanical causes of hip pain. Arthroscopy 2011;27(2):235–51.
39. Leunig M, Beaulé PE, Ganz R. The concept of femoroacetabular impingement: current status and future perspectives. Clin Orthop Relat Res 2009;467(3): 616–22.
40. Clohisy JC, St John LC, Nunley RM, et al. Combined periacetabular and femoral osteotomies for severe hip deformities. Clin Orthop Relat Res 2009;467(9): 2221–7.
41. Naal FD, Miozzari HH, Wyss TF, et al. Surgical hip dislocation for the treatment of femoroacetabular impingement in high-level athletes. Am J Sports Med 2011; 39(3):544–50.

42. Novais EN, Heyworth BE, Stamoulis C, et al. Open surgical treatment of femoroacetabular impingement in adolescent athletes: preliminary report on improvement of physical activity level. J Pediatr Orthop 2014;34(3):287–94.

43. Bizzini M, Notzli HP, Maffiuletti NA. Femoroacetabular impingement in professional ice hockey players: a case series of 5 athletes after open surgical decompression of the hip. Am J Sports Med 2007;35(11):1955–9.

44. Sink EL, Beaulé PE, Sucato D, et al. Multicenter study of complications following surgical dislocation of the hip. J Bone Joint Surg Am 2011;93(12):1132–6.

45. Olson KM, Dairyko GH, Toolan BC. Salvage of chronic instability of the syndesmosis with distal tibiofibular arthrodesis. J Bone Joint Surg Am 2011;93(1):66–72.

46. Espinosa N, Rothenfluh DA, Beck M, et al. Treatment of femoro-acetabular impingement: preliminary results of labral refixation. J Bone Joint Surg Am 2006;88(5):925–35.

47. Botser IB, Smith TW, Nasser R, et al. Open surgical dislocation versus arthroscopy for femoroacetabular impingement: a comparison of clinical outcomes. Arthroscopy 2011;27(2):270–8.

48. Alradwan H, Philippon MJ, Farrokhyar F, et al. Return to preinjury activity levels after surgical management of femoroacetabular impingement in athletes. Arthroscopy 2012;28(10):1567–76.

49. Casartelli NC, Leunig M, Maffiuletti NA, et al. Return to sport after hip surgery for femoroacetabular impingement: a systematic review. Br J Sports Med 2015; 49(12):819–24.

50. Philippon MJ, Weiss DR, Kuppersmith DA, et al. Arthroscopic labral repair and treatment of femoroacetabular impingement in professional hockey players. Am J Sports Med 2010;38(1):99–104.

51. Philippon M, Schenker M, Briggs K, et al. Femoroacetabular impingement in 45 professional athletes: associated pathologies and return to sport following arthroscopic decompression. Knee Surg Sports Traumatol Arthrosc 2007;15(7): 908–14.

52. Sansone M, Ahlden M, Jonasson P, et al. Good results after hip arthroscopy for femoroacetabular impingement in top-level athletes. Orthop J Sports Med 2015;3(2). 2325967115569691.

53. Brunner A, Horisberger M, Herzog RF. Sports and recreation activity of patients with femoroacetabular impingement before and after arthroscopic osteoplasty. Am J Sports Med 2009;37(5):917–22.

54. Nho SJ, Magennis EM, Singh CK, et al. Outcomes after the arthroscopic treatment of femoroacetabular impingement in a mixed group of high-level athletes. Am J Sports Med 2011;39(1 Suppl):14S–9S.

55. Byrd JWT, Jones KS. Arthroscopic management of femoroacetabular impingement in athletes. Am J Sports Med 2011;39(Suppl):7S–13S.

56. Malviya A, Paliobeis CP, Villar RN. Do professional athletes perform better than recreational athletes after arthroscopy for femoroacetabular impingement? Clin Orthop Relat Res 2013;471(8):2477–83.

57. Sing DC, Feeley BT, Tay B, et al. Age-related trends in hip arthroscopy: a large cross-sectional analysis. Arthroscopy 2015;31(12):2307–13.e2.

58. Wenger DR, Kishan S, Pring ME. Impingement and childhood hip disease. J Pediatr Orthop B 2006;15(4):233–43.

59. Philippon MJ, Yen Y-M, Briggs KK, et al. Early outcomes after hip arthroscopy for femoroacetabular impingement in the athletic adolescent patient: a preliminary report. J Pediatr Orthop 2008;28(7):705–10.

60. Tran P, Pritchard M, O'Donnell J. Outcome of arthroscopic treatment for cam type femoroacetabular impingement in adolescents. ANZ J Surg 2013;83(5):382–6.
61. Fabricant PD, Heyworth BE, Kelly BT. Hip arthroscopy improves symptoms associated with FAI in selected adolescent athletes. Clin Orthop Relat Res 2012; 470(1):261–9.
62. De Sa D, Cargnelli S, Catapano M, et al. Femoroacetabular impingement in skeletally immature patients: a systematic review examining indications, outcomes, and complications of open and arthroscopic treatment. Arthroscopy 2015; 31(2):373–84.
63. Leunig M, Beck M, Kalhor M, et al. Fibrocystic changes at anterosuperior femoral neck: prevalence in hips with femoroacetabular impingement. Radiology 2005; 236(1):237–46.
64. Singh PJ, O'Donnell JM. The outcome of hip arthroscopy in Australian football league players: a review of 27 hips. Arthroscopy 2010;26(6):743–9.
65. Crawford K, Philippon MJ, Sekiya JK, et al. Microfracture of the hip in athletes. Clin Sports Med 2006;25(2):327–35, x.
66. McDonald JE, Herzog MM, Philippon MJ. Return to play after hip arthroscopy with microfracture in elite athletes. Arthroscopy 2013;29(2):330–5.
67. Ellis HB, Briggs KK, Philippon MJ. Innovation in hip arthroscopy: is hip arthritis preventable in the athlete? Br J Sports Med 2011;45(4):253–8.
68. Byrd JWT, Jones KS. Hip arthroscopy in athletes 10-year follow-up. Am J Sports Med 2009;37(11):2140–3.
69. Engebretsen L, Steffen K, Alsousou J, et al. IOC consensus paper on the use of platelet-rich plasma in sports medicine. Br J Sports Med 2010;44(15):1072–81.
70. Philippon MJ, Briggs KK, Hay CJ, et al. Arthroscopic labral reconstruction in the hip using iliotibial band autograft: technique and early outcomes. Arthroscopy 2010;26(6):750–6.
71. Ayeni OR, Alradwan H, de Sa D, et al. The hip labrum reconstruction: indications and outcomes–a systematic review. Knee Surg Sports Traumatol Arthrosc 2014; 22(4):737–43.
72. Boykin RE, Patterson D, Briggs KK, et al. Results of arthroscopic labral reconstruction of the hip in elite athletes. Am J Sports Med 2013;41(10):2296–301.

Return to Play Following Anterior Cruciate Ligament Reconstruction

Ryan C. Morris, DO[a], Michael J. Hulstyn, MD[a],
Braden C. Fleming, PhD[b], Brett D. Owens, MD[a],
Paul D. Fadale, MD[a],*

KEYWORDS

- Return to play • Anterior cruciate ligament reconstruction • MRI • Psychology

KEY POINTS

- Validated reliable consensus guidelines are needed to determine when an athlete is ready to return to play.
- The psychological state is the most overlooked factor in evaluating an athlete's return to play, thus, necessitating validated psychological evaluation tools.
- MRI may play a more objective role in the determination of graft health and an athlete's readiness for sport.

INTRODUCTION

Anterior cruciate ligament (ACL) tears are a common sports injury; it is estimated up to 200,000 ACL reconstructions (ACLR) are performed yearly.[1] Oftentimes these ACLR patients were participating in organized sports at a high level before their injury.[2] In athletes, reconstruction remains the optimal treatment to restore knee function.[3] After ACLR and rehabilitation it is estimated that 35% to 60% of patients do not fully return to self-reported preinjury knee function.[4,5]

Return to play (RTP) is an outcome measure for an athlete's ability to perform sports after ACLR. RTP has been reported at 49% to 92% to some level of competitive sport (at or by) 12 to 13 months.[6–8] Unfortunately as few as 33% return to their preinjury level of play.[6–8] Time since surgery was the most often used criterion for RTP after

Disclosure statement: The authors have indicated they have no financial relationships relevant to this article to disclose.
[a] Department of Orthopaedics, Warren Alpert Medical School of Brown University, 2 Dudley Street, Suite 200, Providence, RI 02905, USA; [b] Department of Orthopaedics, Warren Alpert Medical School of Brown University, Coro West, Suite 404, 1 Hoppin Street, Providence, RI 02930, USA
* Corresponding author.
E-mail address: fadalepaul@gmail.com

Clin Sports Med 35 (2016) 655–668
http://dx.doi.org/10.1016/j.csm.2016.05.009   **sportsmed.theclinics.com**

reconstruction.[1] There is limited evidence to support a strict timeline for safe return to sport. Formal objective guidelines are needed to permit safe athletic return.

A second injury of the reconstructed graft or the contralateral ACL seems to be a growing problem. Second injury rates in the general population 5 years after reconstruction are 6.0%,[9] and the rates in younger athletes have been found as high as 29.5%.[10] Fifty percent of these injuries occurred within the first 72 athletic exposures, compared with a 25% injury rate in the control group of pivoting/cutting sport athletes. The concern for reinjury after reconstruction drives a surgeon's thought process for RTP, whereas the athlete may be driven by physical ability.

An athlete may not be able to RTP despite passing all objective criteria, due to their psychological state. A meta-analysis of 5770 patients revealed a 44% return to competitive sport at a mean follow-up of 41.5 months.[6] Eight-five percent to 90% of these patients achieved normal knee function by patient-reported outcomes, objective measurements of knee laxity, and knee strength. A prospective study[8] reported 65% return to the same level of sport activity, even though 90% of patients demonstrated less than 3 mm of side-to-side difference in knee stability by an arthrometer. RTP patients had significantly better scores on a psychological questionnaire and patient-reported outcomes. Despite the apparent success in restoring knee stability and function, there may be a psychological disparity between athletes that RTP and those that do not.

Today, ACLR is more predictable with a shortened timeline for RTP due in part to accelerated rehabilitation that encourages early motion, strength recovery, and return of function.[11] Reconstruction restores knee stability, has high patient satisfaction, and successful outcome measures allowing most athletes to return to an active lifestyle. The ultimate goal of ACLR for the competitive athlete is return to sport. Despite the success and advancements in reconstruction, some athletes still fail to RTP.

RETURN-TO-PLAY DEFINITION

Defining RTP is fundamental as the term allows for multiple interpretations. It is an outcome measure for an athlete's ability to perform sports after ACLR. The time period to allow an athlete to return to unrestricted sporting activity after reconstruction remains controversial. RTP should be defined as the period of time after ACLR at which an athlete competes with other athletes at the same level in official games.

A systematic review of level I randomized controlled trials (RCTs) for published RTP guidelines after ACLR has been performed.[12] Of 49 studies, 90% failed to show objective criteria and 65% listed no criteria for return to sport. The included articles that had a description of criteria for RTP were highly variable and poorly described.[12] Eighty-six percent of studies permitted RTP by 9 months, of which 51% allowed unrestricted RTP at 6 months.[12]

Return to sport does not necessarily require full function. Oftentimes athletes are released to RTP between 6 and 12 months, even though muscle weakness and imbalance can persist for up to 2 years.[13] McCullough and colleagues[2] reported from the Multicenter Orthopaedic Outcome Network (MOON) cohort that only 43% of college and high school players RTP at their self-described performance level. There were 27% that reported they were not at the level before ACL injury, and 30% were unable to play at all.[2] Of athletes who did not RTP within 1 year of ACLR, 91% returned to some form of sport within 2 years. This statistic suggests that some athletes can take longer than the clinically expected time of RTP within 1 year.[14]

RETURN-TO-PLAY RISKS

A recent systematic review and meta-analysis demonstrated RTP placed athletes at a 7% risk for reinjury of their ipsilateral knee and an 8% risk for reinjury of their contra-lateral knee. Athletes younger than 25 years old have a secondary ACL injury rate (ipsilateral + contralateral) of 23% when they RTP to high-risk cutting and pivoting sports.[15] Within 24 months of ACLR there was nearly 6 times greater incidence of a second ACL injury in young athletes after ACLR and return to sport as compared with healthy control participants.[10] The MOON cohort demonstrated that in soccer athletes ACLR on the nondominant limb potentially places the dominant limb at a 16% risk for future ACL injury, whereas ACLR on their dominant limb infers a 3.5% risk to their nondominant limb.[16]

RETURN-TO-PLAY RATES

RTP rates are quite variable depending on the level at which the athlete participates. Shah and colleagues[17] reported a 63% return to sport of professional football players after ACLR, which is consistent with other studies.[2,6,7] McCullough and colleagues[2] demonstrated from the MOON cohort that RTP was 69% for college football players and 63% for high school athletes.[2] In a retrospective cohort study, Division I or I-AA football players, who had undergone ACLR, achieved equal levels of performance with age-, size-, and position-matched controls in National Football League (NFL) com-bined testing.[18] Therefore, high athletic performance is attainable after reconstruction.

National Hockey League hockey players have demonstrated an 81% RTP for one or more full seasons at a mean of 9.8 months.[19] National Basketball Association basket-ball players have shown to have a return to sport of 84.6% and a significant decrease in the number of games played in seasons 1 to 3 years after ACLR, although at 3 years they returned to their preinjury player efficiency rating.[20]

The overall return to sport for National Collegiate Athletic Association Southeastern Conference women soccer players was 85%. There was a statistically significant difference in return to sport rates for athletes in earlier years of eligibility and scholar-ship athletes, 91% versus 46% for nonscholarship athletes. Scholastic standing and individual skill level may be a strong determinant for RTP.[21] Soccer players from the MOON cohort demonstrated that younger and male soccer players were more likely to return to sport after ACLR and that return to soccer declined over time.[16] Patients may frequently shift their priorities because of job demands or family commitments or they move on to a different stage in their life. In patients who are transitioning between high school to university, full-time student to full-time work, and/or single to married life, sports may be absent or no longer be a large part of their lives.[22] These confound-ing variables are oftentimes hard to decipher from the literature and, in turn, falsely decrease the number of athletes that RTP.

Athletes with no previous ACL reconstruction on either knee had more than 4 times increased odds of RTP of their preinjury sport than those with previous reconstruction on either knee.[14] Shelbourne and colleagues[23] showed 74% return to sport at prein-jury level of high school and college athletes and 62% in recreational-level adults after revision ACLR with bone-patellar tendon bone autograft.

FUNCTIONAL TESTING

Isokinetic testing (IT) uses isolated open-chain movements, which are in a single plane of movement. Athletic activities are multiplane and multi-joint in nature consisting of closed-chain movements.[24] IT is useful for assessing a patient's progression through a rehabilitation program but is limited to assess sports performance. Functional movement tests have become the norm for assessing agility, balance, strength, and proprioception that are needed before RTP.

Early activities focus on landing, oftentimes consisting of stepping off of plyometric drill boxes, along with double- and single-leg jumping. A single-leg step-down test (**Fig. 1**) can be used early on to assess the knee extensor group. Qualitative assessment of faulty movement patterns, including contralateral hip drop, ipsilateral hip hike, increased valgus of the knee, and increased plantar flexion of the contralateral foot, can be recognized.[25] When examining the differences in knee, hip, and ankle kinematics, the drop-jump test produced greater knee abduction, possibly designating its importance in evaluating ACL risk in athletes.[25] The vertical drop-jump (VDJ) test has been advocated as a screening tool for ACL injury risk based on knee kinematics and kinetics in a single small sample.[26] Recently medial knee displacement when performing the VDJ test in elite soccer and handball players, who have had previous ACL injury, was associated with an increased risk for contralateral and ipsilateral ACL injury. However, it is interesting that in a cohort of 643 players without previous injury, there were no associations with medial knee displacement on VDJ. Therefore, in this cohort, VDJ cannot be used as a screening test.[27]

The single-leg step-down test produces greater motion in the frontal and transverse planes at the ankle and hip, demonstrating its potential to evaluate control at the hip. Earl and colleagues[25] concluded that the drop jump test and the single leg step-down test should be used together for the evaluation of athletes. It was first reported that dynamic valgus observed during a drop vertical tests was a significant risk factor for ACL injury, reinjury, and contralateral injury.[26,28] Optimizing neuromuscular control of the hip and knee after ACLR, through a decrease in dynamic valgus, may decrease the risk of knee injury following RTP.[28]

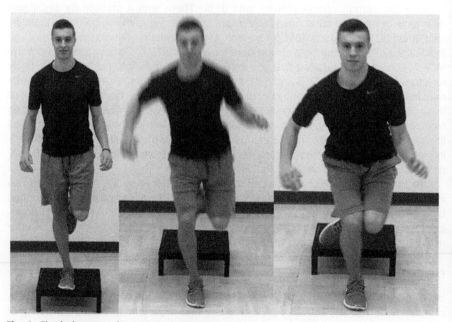

Fig. 1. Single-leg step-down test.

The hop test[29] gauges both strength and confidence in an athletic-based nature and is both a measurement of the return of function level and a perception of knee function.[30] In current clinical practice, the single-leg (**Fig. 2**), crossover (**Fig. 3**), triple, and timed 6-minute hop test are the most commonly used functional assessments.[31] The limb symmetry index (LSI)[32] is the test performance on the operative limb expressed as a percentage of the test performance on the contralateral limb. A recent systematic review[31] encompassing 5000 patients found that most athletes reach 90% LSI at 6 to 9 months after ACLR. The demanding endurance hop testing reflected that there are larger LSI deficits at 6 to 9 months postoperatively, which later normalize at 24 months after reconstruction.[31] Similarly, the single-leg hop test found that two-thirds of patients showed abnormal hop symmetry at 11 months after ACLR, under fatigued conditions, whereas they were normal under nonfatigued conditions.[33] Endurance hop testing may help to elucidate ACLR athletes that need additional

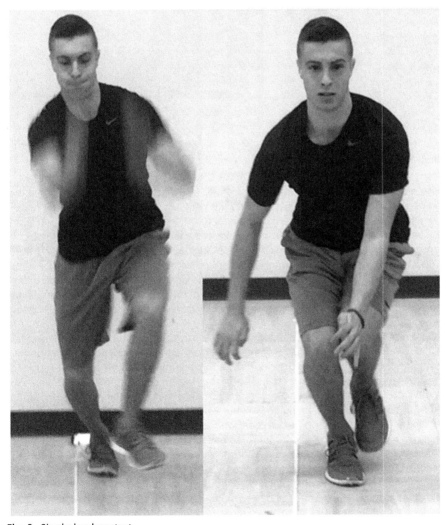

Fig. 2. Single-leg hop test.

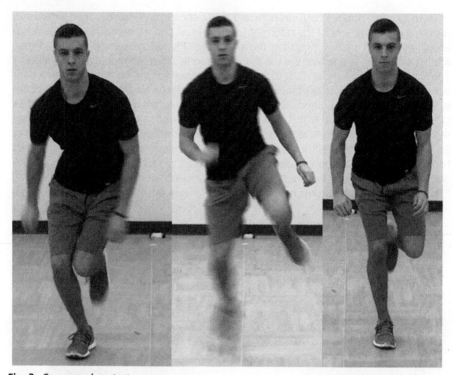

Fig. 3. Crossover hop test.

therapy before RTP, as studies have shown that ACL injuries often tend to occur at the end of a sporting event when participants are fatigued.[33]

IT and unilateral hop testing are often used to make the determination for RTP, but neither have been reported to be predictive of subsequent injuries. Mayer and colleagues[34] used functional tests to compare ACLR patients who were allowed to return to sport with those who were not, based on traditional clinical impairment measures accessing swelling, range of motion, strength, and graft stability. There were no differences in Functional Motor Screen or in the Lower Quarter Y Balance Test functional scores in patients after ACLR that were clinically deemed appropriate for RTP based on clinical criteria.[34]

Gardinier and colleagues[35] used an electromyography-driven musculoskeletal model to estimate joint contact forces and performed RTP readiness testing on patients 6 months after ACLR. The return-to-sport testing consisted of 2 self-reported questionnaires, 4 unilateral hop tests, and isometric quadriceps strength testing. Six months after reconstruction, joint contact force asymmetry on gait analysis predicted failure of return-to-sport testing.[35] Patients who passed RTP testing did not exhibit significant or meaningful contact forces, whereas patients who failed return-to-sport testing exhibited meaningful contact force asymmetries.

Testing in the presence of coaches and/or parents can be advantageous to convey the athlete's ability as opposed to their perception of readiness to RTP. However, the use of functional tests is institution specific as there are no published consensus guidelines to follow. There has not been a single outcome variable that has been correlated with an athlete's ability to RTP. Most clinicians use a combination of clinical examination tests, functional tests, and patient-reported outcomes to determine readiness for sport. Given the lack of a biological-based time point for safe return to sport, the physician is challenged in ascertaining the appropriate time for RTP.

MRI

Magnetic resonance (MR) has been recently used to evaluate the healing process of the ligamentous structures.[36] The linear combination of median signal intensity (SI) and graft volume has been shown to provide a more complete evaluation of the biomechanical properties of the ligament, measured ex vivo, than either variable alone.[37,38] Biercevicz and colleagues[39] established a link between commonly used clinical assessment tools and biomechanical graft integrity by using these MR parameters. The single-leg hop score was predicted at both the 3-year ($P = .008$) and 5-year ($P = .003$) follow-up. At the 5-year follow-up the combination of volume and median SI in a multiple line regression model was also associated with the Knee Injury and Osteoarthritis Outcome Scores (KOOS): KOOS-Quality of Life ($P = .12$), KOOS-Sport ($P = .048$), KOOS-Pain ($P = .017$), and KOOS-Symptom ($P = .021$). Although the KOOS-Activity of Daily Living was not predicted by the 5-year follow-up, this subscore has been shown to indicate patient surgical outcomes the least.[40,41] Larger grafts with lower median SI values (**Fig. 4**) were associated with better knee performance based on traditional outcomes at the 5-year follow-up.[39] Better knee function demonstrated through a higher hop score[32] at a functional outcome at 5-year follow-up tend to have a lower median SI and larger grafts.[39] Patients with higher subscores (indicating better knee function) at 5-year follow-up KOOS divisions of Sports, Pain, Quality of Life, and Symptoms demonstrated larger graft volumes and lower SI scores.[39,40] Research has correlated higher strength or biomechanical properties with lower graft or ligament SI[37,38] and larger graft or ligament volume.[37,42,43] The same MR parameter that relates to graft biomechanical performance was also predictive of overall patient knee health and ACL reconstruction surgical outcomes.[39] Future methods of assessing graft maturity and healing through MRI may become an important clinical assessment tool to determine RTP; with greater understanding of when an ACLR has healed, it may elucidate when a graft may tolerate the forces required for athletic return.

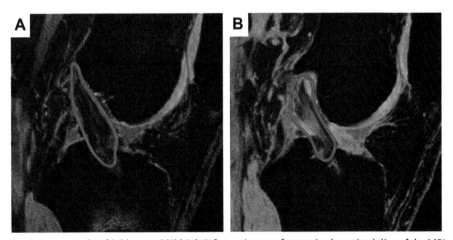

Fig. 4. An example of (*A*) low and (*B*) high SI for patient graft on a single sagittal slice of the MRI stack (*Red lines* outline the ACL graft). (*From* Biercevicz AM, Akelman MR, Fadale PD, et al. MRI volume and signal intensity of ACL graft predict clinical, functional, and patient-oriented outcome measures after ACL reconstruction. Am J Sports Med 2015;43(3):693–9. Figure 4 page 6.)

PSYCHOLOGY

Rehabilitation after injury is difficult for patients. Return to sport depends on both physical and psychological factors. Shah and colleagues[17] reported a 63% RTP for professional football players after ACLR, which is consistent with other studies.[2,6,7] The performance of NFL players that RTP has been shown to be significantly compromised in comparison with preinjury play,[44] despite objective data showing similar performance-based measures in more than 90% percent of athletes.[6]

Kinesophobia, the fear of reinjury, is the most cited psychological variable among athletes for their inability to RTP.[2,6] Patients who were unable to return to preinjury abilities were more afraid of a reinjury as shown by the Tampa Scale of Kinesophobia (TSK).[45] MOON cohort data demonstrated a 43% return to the same performance level among high school and college football players; kinesophobia was the reason cited by 50% of athletes.[2] College athletes who RTP had better patient-oriented outcomes and higher knee-related quality of life than athletes who failed to return to sport.

Patients with good knee function after a primary ACLR who do not return to their preinjury level of sport were largely influenced by individual personalities, shifts in priority, and fear.[22] Patients report multiple types of fear: fear of playing the sport, fear of pain, fear of added financial burden, and fear of being debilitated. Patients who RTP also report being fearful particularly during their initial athletic return, but they were able to overcome this hurdle and relieve themselves of this fear. Both groups reported fear; those that return to sport choose to use their fears as a motivator or barrier to overcome in order to return to sport.

Patient satisfaction has been strongly linked to individual perceptions of symptoms and function.[46] Adherence to rehabilitation protocol after ACLR was a strong indicator of perceived knee function.[47] Patients who attended a higher percentage of therapy sessions reported fewer knee symptoms at 6 months postoperatively.[48] Multiple factors have been shown to affect postoperative compliance (**Table 1**), including self-efficacy[49] and a patient's psychological readiness for surgery[50]; both positively influenced adherence to rehabilitation and outcomes. Self-efficacy is a judgment of one's potential to carry out a task. Self-motivation was identified as the most important factor for compliance with physical therapy protocols.[51] Encouragement through teammates or therapists can help patients complete difficult rehabilitation tasks in undermotivated patients. If patients requiring more encouragement are recognized early during rehabilitation, proper support structure can be used to maximize the rehabilitation benefit.

There are age-related differences in adherence to rehabilitation. Adolescent ACL patients may have hindered rehabilitation due to higher preoperative mood disturbances, instances of pain intolerance, anxiety, and catastrophizing.[52] In those that have a strong athletic identity, success or failure as an athlete can influence

Table 1		
Psychological characteristics that may affect rehabilitation		
Positive	Negative	
High self-efficacy	Low self-efficacy, pessimism, fear of reinjury	
Internal locus of control	External or chance locus of control, threatened athletic identity	
Motivation	Low self-esteem, lack of motivation	
Low anxiety	Anxiety, catastrophizing coping response	

From Christino MA, Fantry AJ, Vopat BG. Psychological aspects of recovery following anterior cruciate ligament reconstruction. J Am Acad Orthop Surg 2015;23(8):501–9.

overall self-worth, motivation, and self-esteem. Therefore, an injury that keeps them from sport can be devastating. Patients undergoing ACLR had a significant decline in their athletic identity with the largest decrease occurring between 6 and 12 months and continued decline over 24 months postoperatively.[53] The 6- to 12-month time period coincides when most athletes are beginning to RTP. During this time period patients may experience anxiety, and their defense mechanisms work to protect their ego. Patients protect their sense of self when their athletic career is threatened or when rehabilitation is progressing slower than expected.[53,54] The time period near RTP for some athletes with high athletic identities may represent a fragile emotional period.

ACL-injured patients are 7 times more likely to have depression compared with the preinjury baseline, along with mood disturbances and lower self-esteem.[55–57] Garcia and colleagues[58] performed a multicenter prospective cohort study in ACLR patients to correlate depression symptoms with patient-rated knee function. They found an overall incidence of 42% major depressive disorder (MDD), and at 1-year follow-up these patients with MDD reported lower mean Lysholm (75.2 vs 88.4) ($P = .04$) and mean International Knee Documentation Committee (IKDC) (71.8 vs 89.3) ($P = .001$) as compared with the non-MDD group. ACLR is an equally effective procedure in patients with MDD and non-MDD patients; however, patients with MDD have statistically significant lower outcomes scores at 1 year postoperatively. Significant mood changes in athletes may persist 6 months after surgery. ACL-injured athletes, as compared with concussed athletes, have reported more emotional disturbances and depression.[55]

Self-efficacy and its implications on ACLR have also been correlated. Thomeé and colleagues[59,60] developed a validated Knee Self-Efficacy Scale and demonstrated high postoperative scores were positively associated with higher activity levels, younger age, male sex, and KOOS outcomes. Preoperative self-efficacy significantly predicted postoperative physical activity, RTP, knee-related quality of life, and single-leg hop test distance 1 year following ACLR.[61] A patient's sense of self-efficacy can play an important role in rehabilitation and outcomes.

The two most important determinants of self-efficacy in ACL-injured patients are patient-reported symptoms and internal locus of control.[60] Those who believe in a relationship between their action and outcome, their internal locus of control, are more likely to have a higher level of self-efficacy. Patients who demonstrated a high internal locus of control scored higher on these subjective outcome measures: KOOS-Activity of Daily Living, KOOS-Sports, and the IKDC Subjective Knee Form.[62] Internal locus of control has been shown to be a predictor of RTP 12 months after surgery.[63]

Ardern and colleagues[63] demonstrated that psychological response contributes to return to sport. More importantly, preoperative and 4-month psychological readiness to RTP demonstrated that fear of reinjury, locus of control, and athlete expectations were found to significantly predict return to preinjury sport abilities at 12 months.[63] When athletes approach return to competition, they may fear letting down teammates and disappointing the coaching staff, loss of fitness after injury, and fear regarding their own performance. The ability to RTP is positively associated with knee-related quality of life and patient-oriented outcomes.

Improving self-efficacy has been a target for psychological intervention. Using modeling videos in a RCT, the treatment group watched videos demonstrating functional tasks, like stair climbing, range-of-motion exercises, and ambulating with crutches.[64] They reported less pain, more self-efficacy, and better IKDC scores postoperatively than the patients in the control group that did not watch the videos.

> **Box 1**
> **Six questions to assess the athlete's emotional vulnerability**
>
> How have you been dealing with your injury/recovery from an emotional standpoint?
>
> Do you feel sad or depressed about your injury/recovery?
>
> Do you feel that you are able to control how well you will do with your rehabilitation?
>
> Do you think you have the mental and physical skills needed to get better?
>
> How are you feeling about yourself at this point in your recovery?
>
> Have you been able to stay involved with your team and teammates?
>
> *From* Christino MA, Fantry AJ, Vopat BG. Psychological aspects of recovery following anterior cruciate ligament reconstruction. J Am Acad Orthop Surg 2015;23(8):501–9.

The ACL-Return to Sport after Injury scale[45] and TSK[65] are validated methods to identify patients' psychological status postoperatively but often are not used clinically. Just taking the time to ask an athlete about his or her emotional state and attitude during recovery can help to determine their psychological state (**Box 1**). This information may help prompt the provider to refer psychological interventions that may improve the athlete's rehabilitation and ultimately his or her outcomes. It is important to pay attention to the psychological issues that may hinder RTP and preinjury abilities as these issues can affect overall patient outcomes.

SUMMARY

The variability in readiness for sport is multifactorial as there is no accepted definition of RTP. Although ACLR procedures continue to be refined, there have been no changes in the recommendations for rehabilitation and/or RTP guidelines. Validated reliable consensus guidelines are needed to determine when an athlete is ready to RTP. The psychological state of athletes must be ascertained so treatment can be instituted that may potentially affect their outcomes. The variability in athletic return may suggest that the ACLR graft is not fully healed and may be unable to tolerate the forces excreted with return to sport. MRI may become an important clinic tool to assess graft maturity and healing, thus, providing the clinician an objective method to determine RTP.

ACKNOWLEDGMENTS

The authors would like to thank Dave Pezzullo MS, PT and Chris Porter for the functional testing images.

REFERENCES

1. Barber-Westin SD, Noyes FR. Factors used to determine return to unrestricted sports activities after anterior cruciate ligament reconstruction. Arthroscopy 2011;27(12):1697–705.
2. McCullough KA, Phelps KD, Spindler KP, et al. Return to high school- and college-level football after anterior cruciate ligament reconstruction: a Multicenter Orthopaedic Outcomes Network (MOON) cohort study. Am J Sports Med 2012; 40(11):2523–9.
3. Frobell RB, Roos EM, Roos HP, et al. A randomized trial of treatment for acute anterior cruciate ligament tears. N Engl J Med 2010;363(4):331–42.

4. Spindler KP, Huston LJ, Wright RW, et al. The prognosis and predictors of sports function and activity at minimum 6 years after anterior cruciate ligament reconstruction: a population cohort study. Am J Sports Med 2011;39(2):348–59.

5. van Eck CF, Schkrohowsky JG, Working ZM, et al. Prospective analysis of failure rate and predictors of failure after anatomic anterior cruciate ligament reconstruction with allograft. Am J Sports Med 2012;40(4):800–7.

6. Ardern CL, Webster KE, Taylor NF, et al. Return to sport following anterior cruciate ligament reconstruction surgery: a systematic review and meta-analysis of the state of play. Br J Sports Med 2011;45(7):596–606.

7. Ardern CL, Webster KE, Taylor NF, et al. Return to the preinjury level of competitive sport after anterior cruciate ligament reconstruction surgery: two-thirds of patients have not returned by 12 months after surgery. Am J Sports Med 2011;39(3):538–43.

8. Gobbi A, Francisco R. Factors affecting return to sports after anterior cruciate ligament reconstruction with patellar tendon and hamstring graft: a prospective clinical investigation. Knee Surg Sports Traumatol Arthrosc 2006;14(10):1021–8.

9. Wright RW, Magnussen RA, Dunn WR, et al. Ipsilateral graft and contralateral ACL rupture at five years or more following ACL reconstruction: a systematic review. J Bone Joint Surg Am 2011;93(12):1159–65.

10. Paterno MV, Rauh MJ, Schmitt LC, et al. Incidence of second ACL injuries 2 years after primary ACL reconstruction and return to sport. Am J Sports Med 2014; 42(7):1567–73.

11. Shelbourne KD, Nitz P. Accelerated rehabilitation after anterior cruciate ligament reconstruction. Am J Sports Med 1990;18(3):292–9.

12. Harris JD, Abrams GD, Bach BR, et al. Return to sport after ACL reconstruction. Orthopedics 2014;37(2):e103–8.

13. Di Stasi SL, Logerstedt D, Gardinier ES, et al. Gait patterns differ between ACL-reconstructed athletes who pass return-to-sport criteria and those who fail. Am J Sports Med 2013;41(6):1310–8.

14. Ardern CL, Taylor NF, Feller JA, et al. Sports participation 2 years after anterior cruciate ligament reconstruction in athletes who had not returned to sport at 1 year: a prospective follow-up of physical function and psychological factors in 122 athletes. Am J Sports Med 2015;43(4):848–56.

15. Wiggins AJ, Grandhi RK, Schneider DK, et al. Risk of secondary injury in younger athletes after anterior cruciate ligament reconstruction a systematic review and meta-analysis. Am J Sports Med 2016. [Epub ahead of print].

16. Brophy RH, Schmitz L, Wright RW, et al. Return to play and future ACL injury risk after ACL reconstruction in soccer athletes from the Multicenter Orthopaedic Outcomes Network (MOON) group. Am J Sports Med 2012;40(11):2517–22.

17. Shah VM, Andrews JR, Fleisig GS, et al. Return to play after anterior cruciate ligament reconstruction in National Football League athletes. Am J Sports Med 2010;38(11):2233–9.

18. Keller RA, Mehran N, Austin W, et al. Athletic performance at the NFL scouting combine after anterior cruciate ligament reconstruction. Am J Sports Med 2015;43(12):3022–6.

19. Sikka R, Kurtenbach C, Steubs JT, et al. Anterior cruciate ligament injuries in professional hockey players. Am J Sports Med 2015;44(2):378–83.

20. Minhas SV, Kester BS, Larkin KE, et al. The effect of an orthopaedic surgical procedure in the National Basketball Association. Am J Sports Med 2016;44(4): 1056–61.

21. Howard JS, Lembach ML, Metzler AV, et al. Rates and determinants of return to play after anterior cruciate ligament reconstruction in National Collegiate Athletic Association Division I soccer athletes a study of the southeastern conference. Am J Sports Med 2016;44(2):433–9.
22. Tjong VK, Murnaghan ML, Nyhof-Young JM, et al. A qualitative investigation of the decision to return to sport after anterior cruciate ligament reconstruction: to play or not to play. Am J Sports Med 2014;42(2):336–42.
23. Shelbourne KD, Benner RW, Gray T. Return to sports and subsequent injury rates after revision anterior cruciate ligament reconstruction with patellar tendon autograft. Am J Sports Med 2014;42(6):1395–400.
24. Abernethy P, Wilson G, Logan P. Strength and power assessment. Sports Med 1995;19(6):401–17.
25. Earl JE, Monteiro SK, Snyder KR. Differences in lower extremity kinematics between a bilateral drop-vertical jump and a single-leg step-down. J Orthop Sports Phys Ther 2007;37(5):245–52.
26. Hewett TE, Myer GD, Ford KR, et al. Biomechanical measures of neuromuscular control and valgus loading of the knee predict anterior cruciate ligament injury risk in female athletes a prospective study. Am J Sports Med 2005;33(4): 492–501.
27. Krosshaug T, Steffen K, Kristianslund E, et al. The vertical drop jump is a poor screening test for ACL injuries in female elite soccer and handball players a prospective cohort study of 710 athletes. Am J Sports Med 2016;44(4):874–83.
28. Paterno MV, Schmitt LC, Ford KR, et al. Biomechanical measures during landing and postural stability predict second anterior cruciate ligament injury after anterior cruciate ligament reconstruction and return to sport. Am J Sports Med 2010; 38(10):1968–78.
29. Daniel D, Malcom L, Stone M, et al. Quantification of knee stability and function. Contemp Orthop 1982;5(1):83–91.
30. Petschnig R, Baron R, Albrecht M. The relationship between isokinetic quadriceps strength test and hop tests for distance and one-legged vertical jump test following anterior cruciate ligament reconstruction. J Orthop Sports Phys Ther 1998;28(1):23–31.
31. Abrams GD, Harris JD, Gupta AK, et al. Functional performance testing after anterior cruciate ligament reconstruction a systematic review. Orthop J Sports Med 2014;2(1):1–10.
32. Reid A, Birmingham TB, Stratford PW, et al. Hop testing provides a reliable and valid outcome measure during rehabilitation after anterior cruciate ligament reconstruction. Phys Ther 2007;87(3):337–49.
33. Augustsson J, Thomeé R, Karlsson J. Ability of a new hop test to determine functional deficits after anterior cruciate ligament reconstruction. Knee Surg Sports Traumatol Arthrosc 2004;12(5):350–6.
34. Mayer SW, Queen RM, Taylor D, et al. Functional testing differences in anterior cruciate ligament reconstruction patients released versus not released to return to sport. Am J Sports Med 2015;43(7):1648–55.
35. Gardinier ES, Di Stasi S, Manal K, et al. Knee contact force asymmetries in patients who failed return-to-sport readiness criteria 6 months after anterior cruciate ligament reconstruction. Am J Sports Med 2014;42(12):2917–25.
36. White LM, Kramer J, Recht MP. MR imaging evaluation of the postoperative knee: ligaments, menisci, and articular cartilage. Skeletal Radiol 2005;34(8):431–52.
37. Biercevicz AM, Miranda DL, Machan JT, et al. In situ, noninvasive, T2*-weighted MRI-derived parameters predict ex vivo structural properties of an anterior

cruciate ligament reconstruction or bioenhanced primary repair in a porcine model. Am J Sports Med 2013;41(3):560–6.

38. Weiler A, Peters G, Mäurer J, et al. Biomechanical properties and vascularity of an anterior cruciate ligament graft can be predicted by contrast-enhanced magnetic resonance imaging a two-year study in sheep. Am J Sports Med 2001;29(6):751–61.

39. Biercevicz AM, Akelman MR, Fadale PD, et al. MRI volume and signal intensity of ACL graft predict clinical, functional, and patient-oriented outcome measures after ACL reconstruction. Am J Sports Med 2015;43(3):693–9.

40. Collins NJ, Misra D, Felson DT, et al. Measures of knee function: International Knee Documentation Committee (IKDC) Subjective Knee Evaluation Form, Knee Injury and Osteoarthritis Outcome Score (KOOS), Knee Injury and Osteoarthritis Outcome Score Physical Function Short Form (KOOS-PS), Knee Outcome Survey Activities of Daily Living Scale (KOS-ADL), Lysholm Knee Scoring Scale, Oxford Knee Score (OKS), Western Ontario and McMaster Universities Osteoarthritis Index (WOMAC), Activity Rating Scale (ARS), and Tegner Activity Score (TAS). Arthritis Care Res (Hoboken) 2011;63(S11):S208–28.

41. Fleming BC, Fadale PD, Hulstyn MJ, et al. The effect of initial graft tension after anterior cruciate ligament reconstruction a randomized clinical trial with 36-month follow-up. Am J Sports Med 2013;41(1):25–34.

42. Fleming BC, Vajapeyam S, Connolly SA, et al. The use of magnetic resonance imaging to predict ACL graft structural properties. J Biomech 2011;44(16): 2843–6.

43. Hashemi J, Mansouri H, Chandrashekar N, et al. Age, sex, body anthropometry, and ACL size predict the structural properties of the human anterior cruciate ligament. J Orthop Res 2011;29(7):993–1001.

44. Carey JL, Huffman GR, Parekh SG, et al. Outcomes of anterior cruciate ligament injuries to running backs and wide receivers in the National Football League. Am J Sports Med 2006;34(12):1911–7.

45. Kvist J, Ek A, Sporrstedt K, et al. Fear of re-injury: a hindrance for returning to sports after anterior cruciate ligament reconstruction. Knee Surg Sports Traumatol Arthrosc 2005;13(5):393–7.

46. Kocher MS, Steadman JR, Briggs K, et al. Determinants of patient satisfaction with outcome after anterior cruciate ligament reconstruction. J Bone Joint Surg Am 2002;84(9):1560–72.

47. te Wierike SC, van der Sluis A, van den Akker-Scheek I, et al. Psychosocial factors influencing the recovery of athletes with anterior cruciate ligament injury: a systematic review. Scand J Med Sci Sports 2013;23(5):527–40.

48. Brewer B, Cornelius A, Van Raalte J, et al. Rehabilitation adherence and anterior cruciate ligament reconstruction outcome. Psychol Health Med 2004;9(2): 163–75.

49. Mendonza M, Patel H, Bassett S. Influences of psychological factors and rehabilitation adherence on the outcome post anterior cruciate ligament injury/surgical reconstruction. N Z J Physiother 2007;35(2):62–71.

50. Udry E, Shelbourne KD, Gray T. Psychological readiness for anterior cruciate ligament surgery: describing and comparing the adolescent and adult experiences. J Athl Train 2003;38(2):167.

51. Pizzari T, McBurney H, Taylor NF, et al. Adherence to anterior cruciate ligament rehabilitation: a qualitative analysis. J Sport Rehabil 2002;11(2):90–103.

52. Tripp DA, Stanish WD, Coady C, et al. The subjective pain experience of athletes following anterior cruciate ligament surgery. Psychol Sport Exerc 2004;5(3): 339–54.

53. Brewer BW, Cornelius AE, Stephan Y, et al. Self-protective changes in athletic identity following anterior cruciate ligament reconstruction. Psychol Sport Exerc 2010;11(1):1–5.

54. Stephan Y, Brewer BW. Perceived determinants of identification with the athlete role among elite competitors. J Appl Sport Psychol 2007;19(1):67–79.

55. Mainwaring LM, Hutchison M, Bisschop SM, et al. Emotional response to sport concussion compared to ACL injury. Brain Inj 2010;24(4):589–97.

56. Smith AM, Scott SG, Wiese DM. The psychological effects of sports injuries coping. Sports Med 1990;9(6):352–69.

57. Morrey MA, Stuart MJ, Smith AM, et al. A longitudinal examination of athletes' emotional and cognitive responses to anterior cruciate ligament injury. Clin J Sport Med 1999;9(2):63–9.

58. Garcia GH, Wu H-H, Park MJ, et al. Depression symptomatology and anterior cruciate ligament injury incidence and effect on functional outcome—a prospective cohort study. Am J Sports Med 2016;44(3):572–9.

59. Thomeé P, Währborg P, Börjesson M, et al. A new instrument for measuring self-efficacy in patients with an anterior cruciate ligament injury. Scand J Med Sci Sports 2006;16(3):181–7.

60. Thomeé P, Währborg P, Börjesson M, et al. Determinants of self-efficacy in the rehabilitation of patients with anterior cruciate ligament injury. J Rehabil Med 2007;39(6):486–92.

61. Thomeé P, Währborg P, Börjesson M, et al. Self-efficacy of knee function as a preoperative predictor of outcome 1 year after anterior cruciate ligament reconstruction. Knee Surg Sports Traumatol Arthrosc 2008;16(2):118–27.

62. Nyland J, Cottrell B, Harreld K, et al. Self-reported outcomes after anterior cruciate ligament reconstruction: an internal health locus of control score comparison. Arthroscopy 2006;22(11):1225–32.

63. Ardern CL, Taylor NF, Feller JA, et al. Psychological responses matter in returning to preinjury level of sport after anterior cruciate ligament reconstruction surgery. Am J Sports Med 2013;41(7):1549–58.

64. Maddison R, Prapavessis H, Clatworthy M. Modeling and rehabilitation following anterior cruciate ligament reconstruction. Ann Behav Med 2006;31(1):89–98.

65. Webster KE, Feller JA, Lambros C. Development and preliminary validation of a scale to measure the psychological impact of returning to sport following anterior cruciate ligament reconstruction surgery. Phys Ther Sport 2008;9(1):9–15.

Return to Play Following Meniscus Surgery

Alaina M. Brelin, MD*, John-Paul H. Rue, MD

KEYWORDS

- Meniscus • Athlete • Sports • Return to play • Repair • Transplant • Meniscectomy

KEY POINTS

- Meniscectomy offers a faster return to play and is a more attractive option to the in-season athlete.
- Meniscus repair should be performed when possible in the young athletically active patient.
- Accelerated rehabilitation protocols for meniscus repair offer equivalent functional outcomes when compared with traditional regimens.
- Meniscal allograft transplantation is a viable salvage procedure, although return to collision or contact sports must be carefully weighed.

INTRODUCTION

The menisci are semicircular, wedge-shaped cartilages that have been identified to play a role in shock absorption, load bearing, and stabilization of the knee. Over the past few decades, an abundance of research has been dedicated to meniscal preservation procedures, as both cadaveric and clinical studies have demonstrated a risk for early degenerative changes in the knee with complete loss of meniscal tissue (ie, total meniscectomy).[1] The vascular supply to the meniscus has also been extensively researched and demonstrates that the outer peripheral third has adequate blood supply (red-red zone), whereas the inner two-thirds tends be more avascular (red-white zone and white-white zone). This has particular implications on the potential healing of a meniscus repair. Knowledge of the zones of blood supply as well as age of the patient and tear characteristics, such as chronicity, tear pattern, and tear location, can aid in making treatment decisions.[2]

MENISCAL INJURIES IN ATHLETES

Studies have suggested that there is an overall incidence of meniscal tears requiring surgery of 60 to 70 per 100,000 person years and approximately one-third of these tears are sport related.[3] Acute traumatic tears are commonly seen in young athletes

Orthopaedic Surgery Department, Walter Reed National Military Medical Center, 8901 Wisconsin Avenue, Bethesda, MD 20889, USA
* Corresponding author.
E-mail address: abrelin@gmail.com

Clin Sports Med 35 (2016) 669–678
http://dx.doi.org/10.1016/j.csm.2016.05.010
0278-5919/16/$ – see front matter Published by Elsevier Inc.
sportsmed.theclinics.com

who are involved in sports that require cutting or pivoting movements.[2] Managing the athlete with a meniscus tear presents a new level of complexity to orthopedic surgeons. There can be significant pressure from coaches, teammates, and athletes themselves to return to play as soon as possible, as lost hours of play can have substantial cost burdens and deleterious consequences to the career of an athlete. With this in mind, the concept of early functional rehabilitation programs has been implemented to provide a faster return to play while still minimizing the risk for reinjury. Nevertheless, the team physician, coach, athletic trainers, and physical therapists must recognize the at-risk player and ensure that rehabilitation protocols are adjusted on a case-by-case basis. Furthermore, rehabilitation will vary depending on the procedure performed and concomitant injuries identified.[4]

MENISCECTOMY

Meniscectomy can involve partial, subtotal, or total removal of the damaged meniscal tissue and should be used only when a repair is deemed infeasible.[5] Factors such as tear type, location, chronicity, and potential to heal should be taken into consideration along with the patient's age when making treatment decisions. When performing this technique, a minimalistic approach should be used when resecting meniscal tissue and a stable rim should remain with a smooth contoured edge to decrease the risk of recurrent tears. Although patients, specifically athletes, are able to return to physical activities much faster following meniscectomy, the risk of early degenerative changes must not be underestimated. A biomechanical study by Lee and colleagues[6] demonstrated that as the degree of meniscectomy increased, the amount of contact stresses across the tibiofemoral joint significantly increased. It is recommended to conserve as much meniscal tissue as possible and to use meniscal-preserving techniques, such as repair, when feasible, especially in patients with high physical demands. Nevertheless, meniscectomy has the benefit of a faster return to activities and sport.

Rehabilitation following meniscectomy typically involves advancing activities as the patient tolerates them. Most are able to return to running, jumping, and sport-specific training at approximately 6 weeks when knee pain and effusions have subsided and quadriceps/hamstring strength has returned to normal. The speed of this program is due to the lack of a healing meniscus, as the damaged tissue has been removed. The standard protocol at our institution progresses in 3 phases: (1) 0 to 2 weeks: begin weight bearing and range of motion as tolerated along with quadriceps, hamstring, and core strengthening; (2) 2 to 4 weeks: addition of sport-specific exercises and return to cardio training; (3) 4 to 6 weeks: continued advancement in sport-specific training and maintenance of strengthening program. The return of full quadriceps function and strength often can be the most rate-limiting step during recovery, so it is prudent to have early strengthening in an athlete's rehabilitation protocol (**Fig. 1**). An athlete is released to competitive sports once equal strength, full range of motion, and endurance in sport-specific exercises has returned, typically within the 4-week to 6-week time frame.

A review of the recent literature demonstrates only a few studies evaluating the return to play of athletes following meniscectomy. An early study by Osti and colleagues[7] evaluated partial lateral meniscectomy in 41 athletes and found that 98% of patients returned to sport at an average of 55 days. When further divided into subgroups, it was noted that patients with an isolated simple longitudinal tear returned the earliest (average 41 days). Kim and colleagues[8] found a significant difference in time to return to play based on age (<30, 54 days; >30, 89 days) and level of competition (elite, 54 days; competition, 53 days; recreational, 88 days). A more recent article by Nawabi

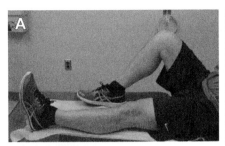
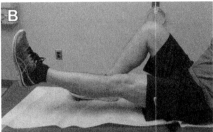
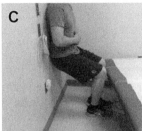

Fig. 1. Quadriceps-strengthening exercises: (A) quad sets, (B) straight leg raise, and (C) wall squat.

and colleagues[9] looking at soccer players undergoing lateral versus medial meniscectomy, identified a shorter time to return to play (5 weeks vs 7 weeks) and a 6.31 higher probability of returning to play in patients undergoing medial meniscectomy as compared with lateral at all time points after surgery. Last, Aune and colleagues[10] evaluated 77 National Football League players, of whom 4 players had midseason lateral meniscectomy and were able to return to play at either 19 or 29 days. It was also noted that speed position players, such as running backs, receivers, linebackers, and defensive backs, were 4 times less likely to return to play.

MENISCUS REPAIR

Meniscus repair remains the treatment of choice for unstable tears in the vascular zone.[11] More recently, in young athletically active patients, the indications are often broadened to include repair of tears extending into the avascular zone of the meniscus. The goal of repair is to maintain as much meniscal tissue as possible so as to avoid alterations in the mechanics of the knee joint and early degenerative changes. Multiple techniques exist for meniscus repair to include inside-out, all-inside, outside-in, and open repair. The inside-out technique remains the gold standard and has been used since the 1980s.[11] The primary disadvantage to meniscal preservation techniques is a longer rehabilitation period, thus further delaying the return of an athlete to sport.

Rehabilitation algorithms for meniscal repair primarily focus on limiting early postoperative weight bearing and deep flexion (>90°). There is a paucity of literature validating postoperative rehabilitation programs; and protocols have largely been anecdotal with very slow progressions and return to sport. Recently, more aggressive approaches have been used with good success and put these traditional methods into question.[12–14] Furthermore, biomechanical analyses provide supportive data that the use of an accelerated protocol is not detrimental to the repair.[15–18] Lin and colleagues[15] demonstrated that compression occurs at the repair site of posteromedial tears with higher flexion angles, thus promoting the use of early, unrestricted range of motion protocols. Additionally, an earlier study showed that partial weight bearing imparted minimal distortion at the repair and advocated for early weight bearing.[16]

Table 1 displays 3 varying accelerated rehabilitation protocols and their outcomes as compared with more restrictive regimens. All demonstrate that accelerated protocols have equivalent functional outcomes. Although earlier accelerated protocol progressions were time-based, Kozlowski and colleagues[19] published a rehabilitation protocol for athletes using a 3-phase progression based on patient abilities. Only the early phase is governed by time so as to protect the repair for the first 6 weeks. Following this, athletes begin a return to sport progression (static, dynamic, and ballistic phases) if they meet specified subjective and objective criteria. The protocol is complete when athletes have full confidence in their knee and once all rehabilitation efforts have been optimized. This algorithm emphasizes the involvement of athletic trainers in the guidance of the rehabilitation and the decision of returning to sport. The protocol used at our institution is displayed in **Box 1**.

Early reports of meniscus repair in athletes proved promising results in this highly active population. DeHaven and colleagues[20] in 1985 reported successful results in 43 of 49 athletes at an average of 5 years by using an open repair technique. Since the advancement of arthroscopic practice, the use of these minimally invasive techniques has largely replaced the historical open methods. **Table 2** provides a comparison of more recent literature on rates and time to return to sport in the athletic population following meniscal repair. This literature exhibits good rates of return to sport in the athletic population following meniscal repair at approximately 5 to 6 months postoperatively.

MENISCAL TRANSPLANT

Meniscal transplant is often viewed as a salvage procedure when minimal viable meniscal tissue remains within the knee and the risk for arthritis progression is high. Although no absolute indications exist, the ideal patient should have undergone a total or near-total meniscectomy and present with joint line pain, mild chondral changes, normal alignment, and a stable knee.[5] Unfortunately, this patient profile can be seen more often than not in the athletic population, as many athletes will incur the risks of in-season meniscectomy for a faster recovery and return to sport.[27] Regarding meniscal allograft transplantation (MAT), there are varying techniques for implantation to include suturing the meniscal allograft to the meniscal remnant or by inserting the allograft with attached bone blocks at the anterior and posterior attachments.[2] Good outcomes will result from appropriate patient selection, proper surgical technique, and the correct postoperative rehabilitation protocol being used.

Postoperative rehabilitation protocols following MAT are similar to that of a large meniscus repair and require significant time away from high-level activities. Heckmann and colleagues[28] in 2006 described their protocol for meniscal allograft transplants. Weight bearing is restricted until 5 weeks. Range of motion begins at weeks 1 to 2 with 0 to 90° and progresses gradually through week 6. Running, cutting motions, and full sports are not instituted until 7 to 12 months postoperatively. This represents a more conservative protocol, which is less desirable for the career-dependent athlete. More recent literature indicates that athletes are being released to full training exercises as early as 4 months postoperatively.[29] Although this is appealing, the treating physician should have a thorough discussion with the athlete on the risks of returning to high-level activities, especially those who partake in collision or contact sports. The rehabilitation protocol that is used at our institution is outlined in **Box 2**. Our

Table 1
Comparison of accelerated rehabilitation protocols following meniscal repair

Article	Weight-Bearing Status	Range of Motion	Exercises	Sport-Specific Activities	Return to Sport	Outcome
Barber,[12] 1994	As tolerated	As tolerated	As tolerated	As tolerated	As tolerated	Accelerated: 90% success rate (vs 81% success rate in standard); not statistically significant
Shelbourne et al,[13] 1996	0–2 wk: as tolerated	0–2 wk: as tolerated	2–4 wk: closed chain resistance, bike, swim	4–8 wk	FROM, operated leg at 75% strength of nonoperated leg	Accelerated: 90% success rate (vs 88% success rate in standard); not statistically significant
Lind et al,[14] 2013	0–2 wk: TTWB 3–4 wk: FWB	0–2 wk: 0–90 3–4 wk: FROM	8 wk: running	No comment	4 mo	Accelerated: 72% success rate (vs 64% success rate in standard); not statistically significant

Abbreviations: FROM, full range of motion; FWB, full weight bear; TTWB, toe touch weight bear.

Box 1
Rehabilitation protocol following meniscus repair

Phase I: 0 to 2 Weeks

- Full wight bearing (WB) in extension
- ± Brace
- Range of motion (ROM) 0 to 90 while non-WB (NWB)
- Isometric quadriceps strengthening

Phase II: 2 to 6 Weeks

- Full WB in extension
- Continue ROM 0 to 90 while NWB
- Add closed chain exercises, terminal knee extensions

Phase III: 6 to 12 Weeks

- Full WB
- Discontinue brace, if using
- Progress to full ROM
- Begin hamstring and proprioception exercises
- Leg press 0 to 90
- Add stationary bike

Phase IV: 12 to 20 Weeks

- Progress with exercises and activities
- Swim at 12 weeks
- At 16 weeks begin sport specifics and run/jump protocol

---

athletes are released to sport specifics at approximately 5 months postoperatively under the guidance of the surgeon, athletic trainer, and coaches. Again, it is emphasized by the treating surgeon that returning to sports can have detrimental effects on the outcome and success of this procedure and, therefore, it is highly recommended to refrain from collision or contact sports.

Although evidence suggests that MAT is effective in relieving pain related to the loss of meniscal tissue, there are limited data on return to sport following this procedure.[27] Noyes and colleagues[30] in 2004 assessed the outcomes of meniscal transplantation in 38 patients younger than 50. Although not specifically evaluating "the athlete," they did identify that 31 of 38 patients were unable to participate in sports activities preoperatively, but at final follow-up (40 months) 29 of 38 patients had returned to higher-level activities to include swimming, biking, running, jumping, pivoting, and cutting. Of note, these patients were not released to light recreational sports until 12 months postoperatively, thus demonstrating a very conservative approach to rehabilitation. A 2010 study by Alentorn-Geli and colleagues[31] reported on 15 soccer players undergoing MAT and followed for an average of 36 months. Of the 14 patients available for follow-up, 12 had returned to play soccer at a mean of 7.6 months. They did not comment on their postoperative rehabilitation protocol. Last, Chalmers and colleagues,[29] in 2013, evaluated 13 athletes who were followed for a mean of 3.3 years after a meniscal allograft transplant. Of these, 10 returned to their previous sport, 9 of whom returned at their desired level of play. Patients were released to full training

Table 2
Comparison of return to sport following meniscal repair in athletes

Author	Number of Patients	Technique	Average Follow-Up	Return to Sport	Average Time to Return to Sport	Average Tegner Score Postoperatively
Mintzer et al,[21] 1998	26 patients (29 repairs); 15 had concomitant ACLR	25 inside out; 4 all inside	5 y	92% returned to sport at preinjury level of activity	Not reported	Not reported
Stein et al,[22] 2009	15 patients	Inside out	2.5 y	Not reported	Not reported	5.9 (vs 6.3 preinjury, not significantly different)
Logan et al,[23] 2009	42 patients (45 repairs); 83.3% of repairs had concomitant ACLR	Inside out	8.5 y	81% returned to preinjury level of activity	11.8 mo for all patients; isolated repair was 5.6 mo	Not reported
Stein et al,[24] 2010	31 patients involved in recreational sports underwent meniscal repair	Inside out	8.8 y	94.4% of repair group returned to their sport at preinjury level	Not reported	5.46 (vs 5.50 preinjury, not statistically significant)
Vanderhave et al,[25] 2011	45 patients (49 knees); 14 patients isolated meniscus repair; 31 underwent concomitant ACLR	Inside out	27 mo	89% returned to preinjury level of activity; 100% of patients undergoing isolated repair (14) returned to full sports	6.5 mo for all patients; isolated repair (n = 14) was 5.56 mo	8 (range 6–9); isolated meniscus repair was 8
Hirtler et al,[26] 2015	37 patients	All inside	24.7 wk	All athletes returned to their sport at preinjury level	27 wk	Not reported

Abbreviations: ACLR, anterior cruciate ligament reconstruction.

Box 2
Rehabilitation protocol following meniscus transplantation

Phase I: 0 to 2 Weeks

- Toe Touch WB brace locked in extension
- ROM 0 to 90 without brace and NWB
- Isometric quadriceps strengthening

Phase II: 2 to 8 Weeks

- 50% WB (weeks 2–4)
- Progress to full WB at 4 weeks
- Brace unlocked 0 to 90 (weeks 2–6)
- ROM 0 to 90 when NWB
- Add closed chain exercises, terminal knee extensions
- All activities with brace; discontinue brace at 6 weeks

Phase III: 8 to 12 Weeks

- Full WB without brace
- Progress to full ROM
- Begin hamstring and proprioception exercises
- Leg press 0 to 90
- Add stationary bike

Phase IV: 12 to 20 Weeks

- Progress with exercises and activities
- Swim at 12 weeks
- Add elliptical

Phase V: More Than 20 Weeks

- Advance to sport-specific activities
- At 16 weeks begin run/jump protocol

---

at 4 months, but it is noted that the average time to return to their previous athletic level was 16.5 months. Overall, this literature demonstrates acceptable results of MAT in the athletic population.

SUMMARY

In conclusion, athletes are a high-demand population, and when treating a meniscal injury, physicians must recognize how surgical decision making and postoperative rehabilitation protocols will affect the athlete's career. Meniscectomy offers a fast return to play with good short-term results, but the long-term risk of osteoarthritis must be weighed when making the appropriate patient selection. Meniscal repair has the benefit of tissue preservation in exchange for a more lengthy rehabilitation, which is less desirable for the in-season athlete. MAT is a sensible option for the athlete with minimal viable meniscal tissue remaining and joint line pain who wishes to maintain an active lifestyle. As the surgeon, one must help the athlete to make a well-informed decision: one that will benefit the athlete's career as well as preserving the health of the athlete's knee.

REFERENCES

1. Belzer JP, Cannon WD Jr. Meniscus tears: treatment in the stable and unstable knee. J Am Acad Orthop Surg 1993;1:41–7.
2. Getgood A, Robertson A. (v) Meniscal tears, repairs and replacement—a current concepts review. J Orthop Trauma 2010;24:121–8.
3. Manson TT, Cosgarea AJ. Meniscal injuries in active patients. Adv Stud Med 2004;4:545–52.
4. Barcia AM, Kozlowski EJ, Tokish JM. Return to sport after meniscal repair. Clin Sports Med 2012;31:155–66.
5. Greis PE, Holmstrom MC, Bardana DD, et al. Meniscal injury: II. Management. J Am Acad Orthop Surg 2002;10:177–87.
6. Lee SJ, Aadalen KJ, Malaviya P, et al. Tibiofemoral contact mechanics after serial medial meniscectomies in the human cadaveric knee. Am J Sports Med 2006;34: 1334–44.
7. Osti L, Liu SH, Raskin A, et al. Partial lateral meniscectomy in athletes. Arthroscopy 1994;10:424–30.
8. Kim SG, Nagao M, Kamata K, et al. Return to sport after arthroscopic meniscectomy on stable knees. BMC Sports Sci Med Rehabil 2013;5:23.
9. Nawabi DH, Cro S, Hamid IP, et al. Return to play after lateral meniscectomy compared with medial meniscectomy in elite professional soccer players. Am J Sports Med 2014;42:2193–8.
10. Aune KT, Andrews JR, Dugas JR, et al. Return to play after partial lateral meniscectomy in National Football League athletes. Am J Sports Med 2014;42: 1865–72.
11. Giuliani JR, Burns TC, Svoboda SJ, et al. Treatment of meniscal injuries in young athletes. J Knee Surg 2011;24:93–100.
12. Barber FA. Accelerated rehabilitation for meniscus repairs. Arthroscopy 1994;10: 206–10.
13. Shelbourne KD, Patel DV, Adsit WS, et al. Rehabilitation after meniscal repair. Clin Sports Med 1996;15:595–612.
14. Lind M, Nielsen T, Faunø P, et al. Free rehabilitation is safe after isolated meniscus repair: a prospective randomized trial comparing free with restricted rehabilitation regimens. Am J Sports Med 2013;41:2753–8.
15. Lin DL, Ruh SS, Jones HL, et al. Does high knee flexion cause separation of meniscal repairs? Am J Sports Med 2013;41:2143–50.
16. Ganley T, Arnold C, McKernan D, et al. The impact of loading on deformation about posteromedial meniscal tears. Orthopedics 2000;23:597–601.
17. Brucker PU, Favre P, Puskas GJ, et al. Tensile and shear loading stability of all-inside meniscal repairs: an in vitro biomechanical evaluation. Am J Sports Med 2010;38:1838–44.
18. Becker R, Brettschneider O, Gröbel KH, et al. Distraction forces on repaired bucket-handle lesions in the medial meniscus. Am J Sports Med 2006;34:1941–7.
19. Kozlowski EJ, Barcia AM, Tokish JM. Meniscus repair: the role of accelerated rehabilitation in return to sport. Sports Med Arthrosc 2012;20:121–6.
20. DeHaven KE. Meniscus repair in the athlete. Clin Orthop Relat Res 1985;(198): 31–5.
21. Mintzer CM, Richmond JC, Taylor J. Meniscal repair in the young athlete. Am J Sports Med 1998;26:630–3.

22. Stein T, Mehling AP, Jost K, et al. Measurements of the quadriceps femoris function after meniscus refixation at the stable athlete's knee. Arch Orthop Trauma Surg 2009;129:1063–9.
23. Logan M, Watts M, Owen J, et al. Meniscal repair in the elite athlete: results of 45 repairs with a minimum 5-year follow-up. Am J Sports Med 2009;37:1131–4.
24. Stein T, Mehling AP, Welsch F, et al. Long-term outcome after arthroscopic meniscal repair versus arthroscopic partial meniscectomy for traumatic meniscal tears. Am J Sports Med 2010;38:1542–8.
25. Vanderhave KL, Moravek JE Jr, Sekiya JK, et al. Meniscus tears in the young athlete: results of arthroscopic repair. J Pediatr Orthop 2011;31:496–500.
26. Hirtler L, Unger J, Weninger P. Acute and chronic menisco-capsular separation in the young athlete: diagnosis, treatment and results in thirty seven consecutive patients. Int Orthop 2015;39(5):967–74.
27. Görtz S, Williams RJ, Gersoff WK, et al. Osteochondral and meniscal allograft transplantation in the football (soccer) player. Cartilage 2012;3:37S–42S.
28. Heckmann TP, Barber-Westin SD, Noyes FR. Meniscal repair and transplantation: indications, techniques, rehabilitation, and clinical outcome. J Orthop Sports Phys Ther 2006;36:795–814.
29. Chalmers PN, Karas V, Sherman SL, et al. Return to high-level sport after meniscal allograft transplantation. Arthroscopy 2013;29:539–44.
30. Noyes FR, Barber-Westin SD, Rankin M. Meniscal transplantation in symptomatic patients less than fifty years old. J Bone Joint Surg Am 2004;86-A:1392–404.
31. Alentorn-Geli E, Vázquez RS, Díaz PÁ, et al. Arthroscopic meniscal transplants in soccer players: outcomes at 2- to 5-year follow-up. Clin J Sport Med 2010;20:340–3.

Return to Play After Medial Collateral Ligament Injury

Christopher Kim, MD[a], Patrick M. Chasse, DPT[b], Dean C. Taylor, MD[a],*

KEYWORDS

- Medial collateral ligament • Partial MCL injury • MCL rehabilitation • Return to play

KEY POINTS

- Grades 1 and 2 medial collateral ligament (MCL) injuries have shown excellent outcomes with nonoperative treatment and adequate rehabilitation. Treatment of isolated grade 3 MCL injuries remains controversial; good to excellent outcomes are reported with both nonoperative and operative treatment.
- Rehabilitation of the injured MCL treated nonoperatively encourages early range of motion (ROM) and progression of activities as tolerated.
- It is possible for athletes with grades 1 and 2 MCL sprains to return to play as early as 1 to 4 weeks from injury. Athletes with grade 3 injuries treated nonoperatively may return as early as 5 to 7 weeks from injury, whereas those whose MCL injuries were treated with surgery may require 6 to 9 months before returning to play.
- Progression to return to play should be criteria based not based solely on timeline.

INTRODUCTION

The MCL is the most commonly injured ligament in the knee.[1] The MCL can be injured in isolation or concomitantly with other structures about the knee. MCL injuries are classified as grade 1, 2, or 3.[2] Grade 1 injuries are microscopic tears of the superficial MCL, the deep MCL, or both. Valgus stress of the knee can elicit pain but no increased laxity. Grade 2 injuries involve partial tears of the MCL, have pain with valgus stress, and may have increased valgus laxity compared with the contralateral side. Grade 3 injuries are complete tears of the MCL and are associated with pain on valgus stress and external rotation, and there is significant valgus instability of the knee. The

Disclosure Statement: Dr D.C. Taylor is the Director of the Duke Orthopaedic Sports Medicine Fellowship. Support for the Fellowship comes from Arthrex, AOA-OMeGA, Breg, DJO, Smith and Nephew, and Synthes-DePuy-Mitek. Dr D.C. Taylor received research support from Histogenics. Dr D.C. Taylor is also a consultant for Synthes-Depuy-Mitek. Drs C. Kim and P.M. Chasse have no disclosures to report.
 a Duke Sports Sciences Institute, Department of Orthopaedic Surgery, Duke University, PO Box 3615, Durham, NC 27710, USA; b Duke Sports Sciences Institute, Department of Physical and Occupational Therapy, Duke University, 3475 Erwin Road, Durham, NC 27710, USA
* Corresponding author.
E-mail address: Dean.Taylor@dm.duke.edu

mainstay of treatment of isolated MCL injuries is nonoperative, especially for grades 1 and 2 injuries. Treatment of grade 3 injuries continues to be controversial. Many are treated nonoperatively whereas others may choose surgery as the initial treatment, depending on injury characteristics.

Given the high incidence of MCL injuries in athletes and their predominant nonoperative treatment, the treating physician should be familiar with common rehabilitation protocols after an MCL injury. A standardized treatment algorithm is difficult to develop, however, perhaps due to the complex anatomy of the medial knee and because MCL injuries are often associated with injuries to a variety of other structures. As a result, the reported rehabilitation protocols vary; prospective comparative studies are limited.[3] Thus, the timing to return to play has also shown variability. Many factors come into play before an athlete returns to sports, including the grade of injury, type of sport, the rehabilitation protocol, and the psychological readiness of the player. Due to this variability in athletes' recovery times, return-to-play decisions should be based on rehabilitation progression and making definitive predictions on time to return to play avoided.

Ultimately, the goal of treatment is returning an athlete to play with no functional limitations and to prevent further injury. This article discusses the treatment, and more specifically, the rehabilitation of MCL-injured athletes and the decision to return to play.

EPIDEMIOLOGY

MCL injuries are the most commonly injured ligament in an athlete's knee.[1,4–7] Injuries may occur from direct contact causing valgus stress or during lateral movements that cause extreme valgus stress on the knee. Common sports where isolated MCL injuries occur include skiing, rugby, football, soccer, and ice hockey. One Australian sports clinic found over a 1-year period that the MCL was the most commonly injured ligament.[5] A recent study of injuries in high school athletes showed that 26% of all ligament injuries to the knee were to the MCL.[7]

Roach and colleagues[8] reported on the incidence of isolated MCL sprains in the United States Military Academy (USMA) from 2005 to 2009. Of the 489 knee ligament injuries, 128 were isolated MCL sprains. The overall incidence rate was 7.27 per 1000 person-years; 73% of injuries were grade 1 sprains, 23% grade 2, and 4% grade 3 sprains. Most injuries (89%) were in male athletes. Male athletes were 2.62 times more likely than female athletes to sustain an MCL injury. A majority of injuries occurred during intercollegiate athletics, including wrestling, judo, hockey, and rugby. MCL sprains are the most common knee ligament injury in professional soccer as well.[9] Lundblad and colleagues[9] performed a prospective cohort study on 27 European professional soccer teams over 11 seasons and recorded 346 MCL injuries, which represented an injury rate of 0.33 per 1000 hours of match play. Almost 70% of all MCL injuries were due to direct contact by collisions, tackling, or blocking. This is in contrast to the anterior cruciate ligament (ACL), where the majority of injuries are due to noncontact mechanisms.

Partial (grades 1 and 2) and full (grade 3) MCL injuries can result in significant time lost rom activities. For example, Roach and colleagues,[8] reported that the median time loss for all grades of MCL injury was 16 days in their study at the USMA. Grade 1 injuries resulted in a median 13.5 days lost, whereas grade 2 and grade 3 injuries resulted in a median 29 days of time lost before being cleared for return to sports. These findings vary slightly from the report by Derscheid and Garrick[10] that focused just on collegiate football players at a single university. Grade 1 sprains lost an average of 10.6 days and grade 2 sprains lost an average 19.5 days. Lundblad and colleagues[9] reported a mean layoff time of 23 days for all grades of MCL sprains in professional soccer players.

It is difficult to quantify a standardized number of days lost before returning to play. There may be variability in grading schemes as well as differences in rehabilitation protocols among treating physicians. In addition, timing is affected by the type of sport and activity to which the athlete is trying to return. Sports, such as hockey or skiing, where the foot and ankle are locked in a boot, place extra stress through the knee and, therefore, may require more time before return. Other sports, such as wrestling, place high rotational forces across the knee during various maneuvers. Although cleared to play, there is also the question of how functional the athlete feels in the early return period. Many athletes return to play with a brace, which may affect performance both physically and psychologically. In addition, there may be a period in which the athlete warms up to playing again and regains the confidence to perform.

MCL injuries typically recover more quickly compared with those of the ACL or posterior cruciate ligament and are thus considered lesser injuries. Most ACL ruptures require reconstruction and players require at least 6 to 9 months before returning to play. Because most are treated nonoperatively, however, the time to return is in the scale of weeks. As such, there is often more pressure on the player and treatment team to define a return time. It is important for the treating physician to be familiar with average return times after an MCL injury; however, return to play should be based on rehabilitation progression, so providers should take care in making predictions on the time to return to play.

PATIENT EVALUATION AND TREATMENT

MCL injuries usually occur after a contact or noncontact valgus stress to the knee. Patients may report hearing a pop and can pinpoint the femoral or tibial location of the injury. There is typically localized swelling and point tenderness. Patients often complain of instability, particularly in the setting of other combined ligamentous injuries.

The initial management of the acutely injured knee includes a thorough physical examination checking for any open wounds and neurovascular compromise. Significant deformity may suggest fracture or dislocation; prompt reduction with immobilization is important. Palpation around the knee, including the entire length of the MCL, helps localize the area of injury. This is important because there are reports of possibly decreased healing potential in distal MCL injuries.[11] Applying valgus stress to the knee at various flexion angles is typically enough to determine the grade of MCL injury. More specifically, valgus stress at approximately 20° of flexion better isolates the MCL. Examination of the knee in full extension allows the cruciate ligaments to contribute to valgus stability.

Rotatory stability can be tested using the Swain test named after the physical therapist J. H. Swain. To perform the test, the knee is flexed to 90° and the tibia is fully externally rotated. The test is considered positive if the patient complains of medial-sided knee pain and may suggest inadequate healing of medial structures, such as the posterior oblique ligament. A positive test also suggests that a player is not ready to return to play.[12]

Imaging should begin with radiographs to rule out fractures or dislocations. Valgus stress radiographs, which show medial compartment gapping, may be useful. Based on a cadaver study, with the knee in 20° of flexion, grade 3 injuries to the superficial MCL show an average 3.2 mm of increased gapping on valgus stress radiographs when compared with the contralateral side. Complete disruption of both the superficial and deep MCL as well as the posterior oblique ligament have on average 9.8 mm of increased gapping versus the uninjured contralateral knee.[13]

An MRI can provide useful information when a high grade MCL injury is suspected. The MRI helps delineate the nature of the injury as well as the location of rupture. Yao and colleagues[14] reported the sensitivity of MRI in diagnosing medial knee injuries as 87%. In grade 3 injuries, an MRI may also show interposition of the pes anserinus between the torn MCL and its tibial attachment. This interposition was described by Lonergan and Taylor as the Stener lesion of the knee, analogous to the interposition of the adductor pollicus aponeurosis seen in thumb ulnar collateral ligament injuries (gamekeeper's thumb). The Stener lesion of the knee is considered an indication for surgery because the interposition of soft tissue may impair healing.[12] Also, MCL injuries are often associated with other knee injuries and an MRI helps rule out other injuries.

Nonoperative treatment has shown excellent outcomes and remains the standard of care for grades 1 and 2 injuries.[15–18] Initial management focuses on controlling pain and swelling with rest, ice, and nonsteroidal anti-inflammatory medications. Emphasis is placed on regaining quadriceps function and knee ROM. Patients are given a brace to prevent repeat valgus stress and to support the leg while quadriceps strength improves. Activity is advanced as tolerated, with early weight-bearing and early initiation of exercises. After a thorough rehabilitation program, athletes may return to play. Patients must demonstrate full pain-free ROM and full strength and state that their knee is stable during activity. The Swain test can be a prognostic measure of when an athlete may begin returning to play. A positive or painful test suggests the patient is not ready. When returning to play, it is highly recommended that athletes wear a functional brace.

Nonoperative treatment of grade 3 MCL injuries can be controversial. Good outcomes have been reported with nonoperative treatment of grade 3 injuries.[17,19–23] Although some clinicians still prefer to begin with several weeks of complete immobilization,[17,24] this has fallen out of favor. Most protocols now encourage early ROM in a brace and a progressive physical therapy protocol. As soon as a patient can tolerate activity, early stationary bike exercises are encouraged and advanced as tolerated. In contrast, side-to- side stress is avoided. Reider and colleagues[23] reported 5-year follow-up results on 35 athletes with isolated grade 3 MCL sprains. Rehabilitation began with ROM exercises in a pool or whirlpool 1 or 2 days after injury. Patients were then given a lateral hinged knee brace to prevent further valgus force with no limits to ROM. The patients were allowed to weight bear as tolerated and immediately began quadriceps setting exercises and straight leg lifts. Overall, athletes were allowed to return to practice when they had achieved full ROM, minimal pain, quadriceps, and hamstring strength within 90% of the uninjured contralateral leg, and the ability to complete a running program (jogging, progressive sprinting, and agility drills). At a mean 5.3 years, all athletes demonstrated good to excellent results.[23] In general, with a proper rehabilitation program, it is possible for athletes to return to full competition approximately 5 to 7 weeks after a grade 3 injury,[25] but as stated, this can be individual and varied.

Surgical treatment may be indicated for athletes with chronic medial instability despite adequate nonoperative treatment and MCL tears combined with other knee injuries. In the setting of an ACL and MCL tear, however, the MCL may still be treated nonoperatively and the ACL reconstructed in a delayed fashion. Some surgeons also recommend surgery as initial treatment of grade 3 injuries, particularly when the MCL fails distally near its tibial attachment.[26–28] As stated previously, the authors recommend surgical treatment of a subset of these distal tears, those with pes anserine interposition — the Stener lesion of the knee.[12]

Surgical treatment consists of primary repair with autograft or allograft augmentation, especially in the acute setting, or reconstruction with an autograft or allograft. Again, initial postoperative management focuses on controlling pain and swelling and regaining quadriceps strength. The patient is given a brace and early ROM is emphasized. Patients often are non–weight bearing initially before progressing to full weight bearing by 4 to 6 weeks. Patients often return to sports 6 to 9 months after surgery.[26–28]

REHABILITATION
Nonoperative Treatment and Rehabilitation

Timelines for return to sport vary and depend on the extent of injury, an athlete's sport and position, associated other injuries, and many other variables. It is possible for patients with grade 1 injuries to return as early as 1 to 2 weeks. It is possible for patients with grade 2 injuries to return in as early as 3 to 4 weeks. The criteria for returning to training and competition include being pain-free with full ROM, no instability on clinical examination, and muscle strength comparable with the uninjured side. Most clinicians want to see the strength of the quadriceps and hamstrings strength at least 90% of contralateral side.[29]

It is possible for patients with grade 3 injuries to return as early as 5 to 7 weeks. Several rehabilitation protocols have been proposed[19,23]; all generally have a satisfactory outcome.[30] Consistent with grades 1 and 2 injuries, timelines for return to sport vary depending on sport and player position.

Staged, criteria-based rehabilitation and return to play are recommended for optimal outcome and should be considered as part of the clinical decision-making model presented in **Tables 1–3** and **Figs. 1–9**.

Operative Treatment Rehabilitation

For an operative patient, the time necessary to return to training and competition is extended because of the surgery. The same staged, criteria-based progression model can be used with postoperative rehabilitation with the addition of healing time considerations and surgeon preferences that are established intraoperatively by the performing surgeon. ROM progression is typically slower than in nonoperative rehabilitation. Typically, full ROM as tolerated begins 4 weeks after surgery. It is ideal to have full ROM at 6 to 8 weeks but may take 6 to 10 weeks to achieve full, pain-free ROM. Lack of progress must be communicated to the surgeon because early manipulation under anesthesia or surgical intervention may benefit patients who have difficulty regaining their ROM.

Scar tissue formation undoubtedly occurs not only at the incision site but also throughout the surgical area. Rehabilitation in the first stage is specific to the operative patient, but the remainder of the rehabilitation program can follow the same outlined phases described for nonoperative rehabilitation.

Rehabilitation in phases 2 and 3 is similar to that in nonoperative patients, but there are several other qualifications for operative patients (presented in **Tables 4** and **5**). As with all surgical patients, proper communication between the surgeon and rehabilitation provider is crucial for appropriate ROM, ambulation, and wound care guidelines.

Consistent with an MCL injury managed nonoperatively, a staged, criteria-based rehabilitation model is recommended for optimal outcome and should be considered

Table 1
Phase 1 rehabilitation for the nonoperative patient (acute phase)

Goal	Rehabilitation Intervention	Comment
Protect injury and promote healing	Brace	Currently no consensus in the literature about bracing but a longer hinged brace is commonly used early in the rehabilitation process and when returning to sports during the same competitive season[24] (see **Fig. 1**). Many prescribe a brace to prevent further valgus stress and until quadriceps function is optimal and the patient can achieve normal gait.
	Rest	—
	Education on avoiding valgus mechanism	Education on strategies to avoid reaggravation of the injury is a crucial part of early rehabilitation. The athlete must understand what a valgus load on the knee is and how this force is applied during activities of daily living. A practical example of this valgus mechanism occurs when dragging one's foot during the initial swing phase of gait (see **Fig. 2**).
Limit inflammation and swelling	Cryotherapy methods	Many methods exist, including but not limited to, cold whirlpool immersion, ice, ice cup massage, Game Ready device, and cryochamber device.
	Elastic compression wraps	—
	Anti-inflammatory medications	—
	Elevation	—
	Modalities	Many methods exist, including but not limited to, neuromuscular electrical stimulation, laser therapy, ultrasound, and compressive units like NormaTec.
Regain ROM and muscle activation	Progress motion as tolerated	—
	Passive ROM → active-assisted ROM → active ROM exercises	—
	Stationary bike	Early ROM using a stationary bike is believed to promote healing of the MCL similar to that of animal models using continuous passive motion devices.[25]
Normalize gait	Gait training	—
	Aquatic therapy	Gait training can begin in water for athletes who present with an antalgic gait. Properties of water that can be beneficial for gait training are seen below.
Advance to next phase	—	Once criteria are met (see **Fig. 3**), the rehabilitation may progress to phase 2

Table 2
Phase 2 rehabilitation for the nonoperative patient (motor control phase)

Goal	Rehabilitation Interventions	Comments
Regain strength	Strengthening exercises (open chain → closed chain)	Progressively strengthen Dynamic knee stabilizers (quadriceps, hamstring) Lower extremity stabilizers above and below the knee (pelvic stabilizers, gluteals, gastrocnemius, soleus) Advance weight bearing as tolerated Isometric → isotonic → eccentric
Address causative factors	Variable	Seek to identify causative factors for the specific type of injury. Treatment and rehabilitation should include prevention strategies to avoid future repeat injuries. Examples of causative factors include weak hip abductors and external rotators, foot pronation and genu valgus postural abnormalities (see **Fig. 4**), increased Q-angle, and weak core musculature. Abnormal body mechanics with sport-specific activities (see **Fig. 5**)
Straight line jogging	Aquatic therapy, treadmill training, grass or turf training	Track symptoms as running progresses Initially maybe beneficial to focus on sport-specific distances, that is, 40-yard jog for football players, then increase speed as tolerated. Methods to address an athlete demonstrating symptomatic or asymmetrical running after injury include aquatic therapy, deep-well jogging with aqua jogger, and harness-supported treadmill. Rapid walking program progressed to run/walk intervals
Advance to next phase	—	Once criteria are met (see **Fig. 6**), rehabilitation may advance to phase 3

Table 3
Phase 3 rehabilitation for the nonoperative patient (return-to-sport phase)

Goal	Rehabilitation Interventions	Comments
Progress jog to sprint	Aquatic therapy, treadmill training, grass or turf training	Similar to phase 2. Focus on distance required by the sport first, then gradually progress repetitions and speed.
Incorporate functional training	Proprioception exercises, agility training, plyometric training, sport-specific training	Plyometric exercises (see **Fig. 7**), agility training (see **Fig. 8**) Introduce exercises specific to the athlete's sport while addressing potential causes of repeat injury such as poor landing mechanics
Assess physical performance	Variable	Physical performance tests (see section Controversies in Return to Sport) Report persistent symptoms with sporting movements to the physician because these may require further evaluation and treatment
Return to sport	—	General criteria to return to sports can be seen in **Fig. 9**.

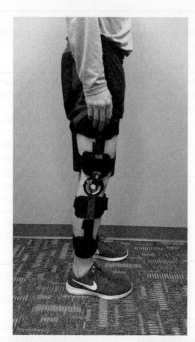

Fig. 1. Long leg hinged brace.

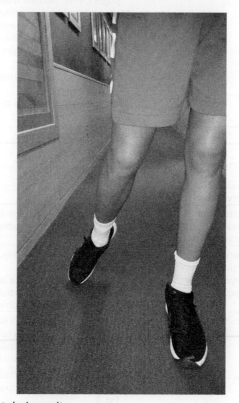

Fig. 2. Dragging foot during gait.

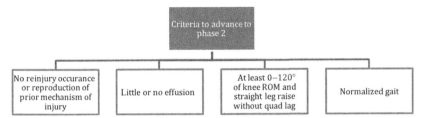

Fig. 3. Criteria to advance to phase 2.

as part of the clinical decision-making model presented in **Tables 4–6** and **Figs. 4, 5,** and **7–10**.

Controversies in Return to Sport

Many controversies exist regarding treatment of isolated MCL injuries, including

- Bracing
  - There is lack of evidence as to whether or not bracing the injured lower extremity prevents further injury in the scenario of isolated MCL injuries.
  - Typically, a long hinged brace is discontinued and a functional athletic brace is used during return to sports (**Fig. 11**).

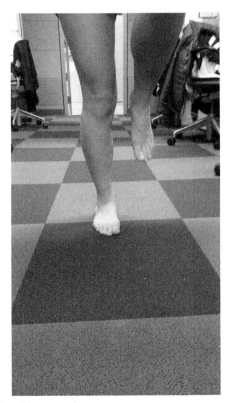

Fig. 4. Pes planus with mild genu valgum.

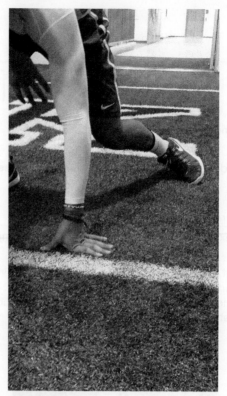

Fig. 5. Abnormal body mechanics.

- Physical performance tests
  - Many physical performance tests have been proposed as objective criteria to return to sports after knee and lower extremity injuries
  - The following tests have been proposed, but there is no consensus or standard across all sports:
    - Isokinetic testing
    - Functional movement screen
    - Selective functional movement assessment
    - Y-balance test
    - Triple-hop test
    - Landing error scoring system

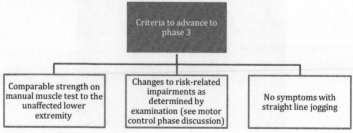

Fig. 6. Criteria to advance to phase 3.

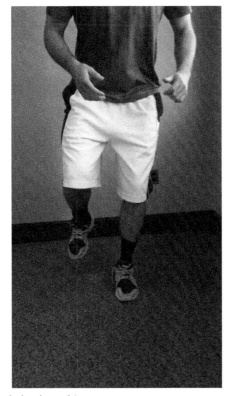

Fig. 7. Plyometrics single-leg lateral jump.

- Timelines versus criteria-based progressions
  - Timelines may be more important during the early phases of postoperative rehabilitation but may not be as important in nonoperative rehabilitation.
  - Nonoperative rehabilitation varies in length and is more effectively designed with criteria for advancement than timelines alone.

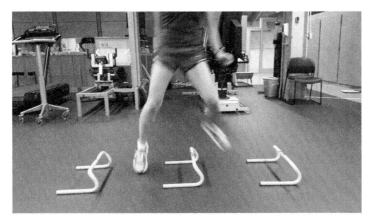

Fig. 8. Agility-training lateral hurdles.

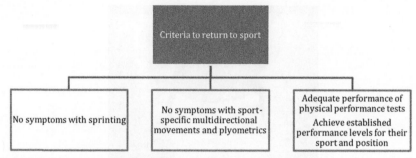

Fig. 9. Criteria to return to sport.

OUTCOMES OF MEDIAL COLLATERAL LIGAMENT INJURY TREATMENT
Nonoperative Treatment

The outcomes of nonoperative treatment of grades 1 and 2 injuries are consistently good to excellent. Patients have been reported to return to play with good function[10,31,32] and most clinicians agree that nonoperative treatment is the standard of

Table 4
Phase 2 rehabilitation for the operative patient (motor control phase)

Goal	Rehabilitation Interventions	Comments

Regain strength[a]	Strengthening exercises (open chain →closed chain)	Progressively strengthen
		  Dynamic knee stabilizers (quadriceps, hamstring)
		  Lower extremity stabilizers above and below the knee (pelvic stabilizers, gluteals, gastrocnemius, soleus)
		  Closed kinetic chain strengthening typically after 6 wk if symptoms and quadriceps control allow
		  Double leg press maybe limited to 70° early on
		Advance weight bearing as tolerated
		Isometric→isotonic→eccentric

Address causative factors	Variable	Seek to identify causative factors for the specific type of injury. Treatment and rehabilitation should include prevention strategies to avoid future repeat injuries. Examples of causative factors include weak hip abductors and external rotators, foot pronation and genu valgus postural abnormalities (see **Fig. 4**), increased Q-angle, and weak core musculature. Abnormal body mechanics with sport-specific activities (see **Fig. 5**)
Straight line jogging	Aquatic therapy, treadmill training, grass or turf training	Track symptoms as running progresses. Initially may be beneficial to focus on sport-specific distances, that is, 40-yard jog for football players, then increase speed as tolerated Methods to address an athlete demonstrating symptomatic or asymmetrical running after injury include aquatic therapy, deep-well jogging with aqua jogger, and harness-supported treadmill. Rapid walking program progressed to run/walk intervals

[a] Strengthening is more gradual in than nonoperative scenario and phase 2 expected to be longer in a postoperative rehabilitation.

Table 5
Phase 3 rehabilitation for the operative patient (return-to-sport phase)

Goal	Rehabilitation Interventions	Comments
Progress jog to sprint	Aquatic therapy, treadmill training, grass or turf training	Similar to phase 2. Focus on distance required by the sport first. Then gradually progress repetitions and speed
Incorporate functional training	Proprioception exercises, agility training, plyometric training, sport-specific training	Plyometric exercises (see **Fig. 7**). Plyometrics typically allowed by 16 wk postoperatively.[30] Must be cautious and observe for symptoms and effusion Agility training (see **Fig. 8**) Introduce exercises specific to the athlete's sport while addressing potential causes of repeat injury, such as poor landing mechanics.
Assess physical performance	Variable	Physical performance tests (see section Controversies in Return to Sport) Report persistent symptoms with sporting movements to the physician as these may require further evaluation and treatment

The return-to-sport criteria for the surgical patient is the same as for the patient treated nonoperatively (see **Fig. 9**).

care for partial MCL injuries.[10,31–33] Lundberg and Messner[32] reported on 38 patients with partial MCL tears, with 74% regaining nearly normal knee function by 3 months. At 10 years' follow-up, 71% had excellent and 92% had good to excellent Lysholm functional scores. At 10 years, however, 13% of patients demonstrated radiographic evidence of early arthritis.[32] An earlier report by Derscheid and Garrick[10] found, over a 4-year period, that 51 of 70 (73%) knee injuries in college football players were grades 1 and 2 injuries. Treatment was rest and early rehabilitation and players returned to play on average 10.6 days and 19.5 days after grades 1 and 2 injuries, respectively.

Nonoperative treatment of grade 3 injuries remains controversial with some showing excellent outcomes[23] and others reporting chronic medial laxity and arthritis.[18,23,31] Reider and colleagues[23] reported the results of early functional rehabilitation on 35 athletes with grade 3 MCL ruptures. Rehabilitation began with early ROM in a pool. Once 90° of flexion was obtained, strengthening exercises were begun. Athletes were allowed to return to practice when they achieved full ROM, minimal pain, quadriceps and hamstring strength within 90% of the other leg, and the ability to complete a running program. At a mean 5.3 years' follow-up, the 50-point Hospital for Special Surgery knee rating score was 45.9, which was comparable to operative treatment. Half of the football players within the group returned to competition within 2 weeks, whereas 16 of 19 returned within 5 weeks. Many athletes, however, required 2 to 4 months before feeling as if their knee returned to full function; the reinjury rate was 3%.

Operative Treatment

Some clinicians have argued that grade 3 MCL injuries may do better with surgical treatment. For example, Kannus and colleagues[31] reported greater instability with nonoperative treatment as well as lower functional scores and higher rates of osteoarthritis on radiographs. Although the initial treatment of isolated MCL ruptures remains controversial, there are certain situations where most surgeons would agree that surgical treatment is preferred. Some clinicians argue that MCL ruptures distally

Table 6
Phase 1 rehabilitation for the operative patient (acute phase)

Goal	Rehabilitation Interventions	Comments
ROM	—	It is crucial to establish a safe zone during initial rehabilitation, commonly 0–90° of flexion for the first 4 wk. These zones are important to avoid arthrofibrosis and soft tissue adhesions.
		Patellar mobilization, soft tissue mobilization (instrument-assisted soft tissue mobilization), and scar tissue mobilization (use modalities [ie, laser, ultrasound] to promote healing and scar tissue removal) are used to improve ROM.[30]
		Progress from passive ROM (usually the first 2 wk) → active assisted ROM → active ROM
		Exercise bike can be used as passive ROM, active assisted ROM, or active ROM.
Ambulation	—	Typically non–weight bearing to touch-down weight bearing, in a long hinged knee brace and axillary crutches for 6 wk (may vary depending on surgeon).
		Gait training should not include aquatic therapy specific interventions until the wound is fully closed
Wound care	—	Observe and assess for signs of infection at every visit Dressings and sutures
		Most surgeons have the athlete return to have sutures removed 10–14 d postoperatively, but the rehabilitation provider is responsible for addressing wound care complications like changing dressings, notifying surgeon or physician assistant of signs of infection, and providing instructions for activities of daily living.
Pain and swelling control	—	Similar to phase 1 of the nonoperative rehabilitation program
		May be increased postoperatively compared with nonoperative
Early strengthening[a]	Quad sets	—
	Straight leg raises	In the brace until the athlete can achieve a straight leg raise without a quad lag)
	Hip abduction/ adduction, extensions	In the brace
	Ankle pumps	Throughout the day
Advance to next phase	—	Once criteria are met (see **Fig. 10**), rehabilitation may advance to phase 2.

[a] Likely more atrophy in muscles compared with nonoperative scenario (especially quadriceps and gastrocnemius).

along the tibia, especially when the pes anserinus is flipped between the MCL and bone (the Stener lesion of the knee[12]), do not heal well with nonoperative treatments.[3] MCL ruptures in the setting of other concomitant injuries, such as a posteromedial corner injury, may also show poor results with nonoperative treatments. In 1983, Hughston and Barrett[34] showed in their case series that 94% of athletes with MCL and associated anteromedial rotatory instability were able to return to their preinjury

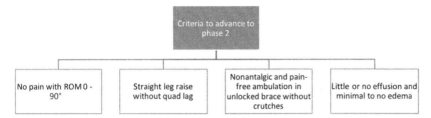

Fig. 10. Criteria to advance to phase 2.

level of athletic function after surgical repair. Eleven years later, Hughston reinforced his earlier findings by again showing overall excellent short-term and long-term results and only a 7% rerupture rate after acute repair of the MCL.[20]

Overall, excellent outcomes have been achieved with nonoperative treatment of grades 1 and 2 MCL injuries.[10,31,32] Grade 3 MCL ruptures have been reported to do well with both nonoperative and operative treatments. Some surgeons argue that grade 3 MCL ruptures treated without surgery do just as well as those treated with surgery.[35] Although short-term results may be promising, there are long-term results that suggest increased risk of instability, ACL insufficiency, and osteoarthritis.[18,23,31]

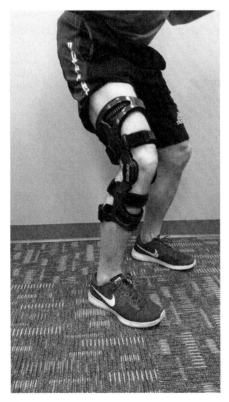

Fig. 11. Functional brace.

SUMMARY AND DISCUSSION

The MCL is the most commonly injured ligament in the knee. Athletes sustain varying severities of injury and this affects their treatment and rehabilitation. A majority of MCL injuries are considered partial (grades 1 and 2). The mainstay of treatment is nonoperative, with emphasis on early ROM and functional rehabilitation. Grade 3 injuries are also treated nonoperatively, but there are conditions where surgery may be the preferred initial treatment. In the setting of chronic instability or a multiligament knee injury, many surgeons manage the ruptured MCL surgically.

The rehabilitation process has evolved for both the nonoperative and operative treatments of MCL injuries. Although some clinicians still prefer complete immobilization in the early period, there has been a shift to early ROM and early functional rehabilitation. This has produced excellent results. The burning question for any young athlete who has sustained an injury is return to play, which remains controversial. There are multiple factors to be considered, including the severity of injury, type of sport, and the rehabilitation protocol. Most people, including patient, parents, coaching staff, agents, and media, think in terms of a timeline. In this regard, there are average timelines that have been reported. In many respects, the treating physician and therapist often progress the rehabilitation according to time from injury or time from surgery. It is also important, however, to consider an athlete's ROM, strength, and function as criteria to progress to eventual return to play. Therefore, the often quoted 1 to 4 weeks for partial MCL injuries and 5 to 7 weeks for complete MCL ruptures treated nonoperatively are simply guidelines and goals for rehabilitation. Likewise, when a patient is told 6 to 9 months before returning to sports after a reconstruction, this too should be used as a guideline, with the understanding that ultimately it is the athlete's function and return of confidence that return them to play.

ACKNOWLEDGMENTS

The authors acknowledge Donald T. Kirkendall, ELS (a contracted medical editor), for his assistance in the preparation of this article.

REFERENCES

1. Miyasaka KC, Daniel DM, Stone ML. The incidence of knee ligament injuries in the general population. Am J Knee Surg 1991;4:3–8.
2. Bergfeld J. Symposium: functional rehabilitation of isolated medial collateral ligament sprains. First-, second-, and third-degree sprains. Am J Sports Med 1979; 7(3):207–9.
3. Smyth MP, Koh JL. A review of surgical and nonsurgical outcomes of medial knee injuries. Sports Med Arthrosc 2015;23(2):e15–22.
4. Baquie P, Brukner P. Injuries presenting to an Australian sports medicine centre: a 12-month study. Clin J Sport Med 1997;7(1):28–31.
5. Chen L, Kim PD, Ahmad CS, et al. Medial collateral ligament injuries of the knee: current treatment concepts. Curr Rev Musculoskelet Med 2008;1(2):108–13.
6. Moore O, Cloke DJ, Avery PJ, et al. English Premiership Academy knee injuries: lessons from a 5 year study. J Sports Sci 2011;29(14):1535–44.
7. Shea KG, Grimm NL, Ewing CK, et al. Youth sports anterior cruciate ligament and knee injury epidemiology: who is getting injured? In what sports? When? Clin Sports Med 2011;30(4):691–706.
8. Roach CJ, Haley CA, Cameron KL, et al. The epidemiology of medial collateral ligament sprains in young athletes. Am J Sports Med 2014;42(5):1103–9.

9. Lundblad M, Walden M, Magnusson H, et al. The UEFA injury study: 11-year data concerning 346 MCL injuries and time to return to play. Br J Sports Med 2013; 47(12):759–62.

10. Derscheid GL, Garrick JG. Medial collateral ligament injuries in football. Nonoperative management of grade I and grade II sprains. Am J Sports Med 1981;9(6): 365–8.

11. Frank CB, Loitz BJ, Shrive NG. Injury location affects ligament healing. A morphologic and mechanical study of the healing rabbit medial collateral ligament. Acta Orthop Scand 1995;66(5):455–62.

12. Lonergan KT, Taylor DC. Medial collateral ligament injuries of the knee: an evolution of surgical reconstruction. Tech Knee Surg 2002;1(2):137–45.

13. Laprade RF, Bernhardson AS, Griffith CJ, et al. Correlation of valgus stress radiographs with medial knee ligament injuries: an in vitro biomechanical study. Am J Sports Med 2010;38(2):330–8.

14. Yao L, Dungan D, Seeger LL. MR imaging of tibial collateral ligament injury: comparison with clinical examination. Skeletal Radiol 1994;23(7):521–4.

15. Halinen J, Lindahl J, Hirvensalo E, et al. Operative and nonoperative treatments of medial collateral ligament rupture with early anterior cruciate ligament reconstruction: a prospective randomized study. Am J Sports Med 2006;34(7): 1134–40.

16. Holden DL, Eggert AW, Butler JE. The nonoperative treatment of grade I and II medial collateral ligament injuries to the knee. Am J Sports Med 1983;11(5): 340–4.

17. Indelicato PA. Non-operative treatment of complete tears of the medial collateral ligament of the knee. J Bone Joint Surg Am 1983;65(3):323–9.

18. Indelicato PA, Hermansdorfer J, Huegel M. Nonoperative management of complete tears of the medial collateral ligament of the knee in intercollegiate football players. Clin Orthop Relat Res 1990;(256):174–7.

19. Ballmer PM, Jakob RP. The non operative treatment of isolated complete tears of the medial collateral ligament of the knee. A prospective study. Arch Orthop Trauma Surg 1988;107(5):273–6.

20. Hughston JC. The importance of the posterior oblique ligament in repairs of acute tears of the medial ligaments in knees with and without an associated rupture of the anterior cruciate ligament. Results of long-term follow-up. J Bone Joint Surg Am 1994;76(9):1328–44.

21. Hughston JC, Eilers AF. The role of the posterior oblique ligament in repairs of acute medial (collateral) ligament tears of the knee. J Bone Joint Surg Am 1973;55(5):923–40.

22. Lind M, Jakobsen BW, Lund B, et al. Anatomical reconstruction of the medial collateral ligament and posteromedial corner of the knee in patients with chronic medial collateral ligament instability. Am J Sports Med 2009;37(6):1116–22.

23. Reider B, Sathy MR, Talkington J, et al. Treatment of isolated medial collateral ligament injuries in athletes with early functional rehabilitation. A five-year follow-up study. Am J Sports Med 1994;22(4):470–7.

24. Hastings DE. The non-operative management of collateral ligament injuries of the knee joint. Clin Orthop Relat Res 1980;(147):22–8.

25. Wijdicks CA, Griffith CJ, Johansen S, et al. Injuries to the medial collateral ligament and associated medial structures of the knee. J Bone Joint Surg Am 2010;92(5):1266–80.

26. Fanelli GC, Harris JD. Surgical treatment of acute medial collateral ligament and posteromedial corner injuries of the knee. Sports Med Arthrosc 2006;14(2): 78–83.
27. Jacobson KE, Chi FS. Evaluation and treatment of medial collateral ligament and medial-sided injuries of the knee. Sports Med Arthrosc 2006;14(2):58–66.
28. Tibor LM, Marchant MH, Taylor DC, et al. Management of medial-sided knee injuries, part 2 posteromedial corner. Am J Sports Med 2010;39(6):1332–40.
29. Marchant MH, Tibor LM, Sekiya JK, et al. Management of medial-sided knee injuries, part 1 medial collateral ligament. Am J Sports Med 2010;39(5):1102–13.
30. Laprade RF, Wijdicks CA. The management of injuries to the medial side of the knee. J Orthop Sports Phys Ther 2012;42(3):221–33.
31. Kannus P. Long-term results of conservatively treated medial collateral ligament injuries of the knee joint. Clin Orthop Relat Res 1988;(226):103–12.
32. Lundberg M, Messner K. Long-term prognosis of isolated partial medial collateral ligament ruptures. A ten-year clinical and radiographic evaluation of a prospectively observed group of patients. Am J Sports Med 1996;24(2):160–3.
33. Fetto JF, Marshall JL. Medial collateral ligament injuries of the knee: a rationale for treatment. Clin Orthop Relat Res 1978;(132):206–18.
34. Hughston JC, Barrett GR. Acute anteromedial rotatory instability. Long-term results of surgical repair. J Bone Joint Surg Am 1983;65(2):145–53.
35. Sandberg R, Balkfors B, Nilsson B, et al. Operative versus non-operative treatment of recent injuries to the ligaments of the knee. A prospective randomized study. J Bone Joint Surg Am 1987;69(8):1120–6.

Return to Play Following Ankle Sprain and Lateral Ligament Reconstruction

Scott B. Shawen, MD[a,b,*], Theodora Dworak, MD[c],
Robert B. Anderson, MD[b]

KEYWORDS

- Return to play • Ankle sprain • Ankle stabilization surgery • Ankle instability
- Syndesmosis injury

KEY POINTS

- Ankle sprains are the most common musculoskeletal injury in athletes.
- Treatment should consist of activity modification and pain control with transition to early range of motion and functional rehabilitation to allow for quicker return to function and decreased reinjury rates.
- Patients with functional or mechanical instability that do not improve with rehabilitation or preventative measures should be considered for operative reconstruction of the lateral ligaments to prevent chronic degeneration, dysfunction, or deformity.
- Concurrent findings, such as osteochondral injury, peroneal tendon injury, loose bodies, impingement, and tarsal coalition, should be considered in patients with continued ankle pain. Advanced imaging with MRI and arthroscopy are tools to further evaluate these concurrent injuries.
- Athletes should return to play only after range of motion and strength of the injured extremity has returned. Athletes with history of prior ankle sprain should be prophylactically treated with either taping or bracing during participation in sport to prevent further and repetitive injury.

INTRODUCTION

Ankle sprains and lateral ankle instability are exceedingly common injuries. However, the incidence of injury varies depending on the activity level of the studied population. These injuries occur most often during axial loading of the foot with inversion stress and a plantar-flexed foot.[1] Subsequent repeat ankle sprain or improper rehabilitation

The views expressed in this article are those of the author and do not reflect the official policy of the Department of Army/Navy/Air Force, Department of Defense, or US Government.
[a] Uniformed Services University of the Health Sciences, Bethesda, MD, USA; [b] OrthoCarolina Foot & Ankle Institute, 2001 Vail Avenue, Suite 200B, Charlotte, NC 28207, USA; [c] Department of Orthopaedic Surgery, Walter Reed National Military Medical Center, 8901 Rockville Pike, Bethesda, MD 20889, USA
* Corresponding author.
E-mail address: scott.b.shawen@gmail.com

following initial injury can result in lateral ankle instability in up to 20% of patients.[2-4] Instability is either functional or mechanical in nature. Functional lateral ankle instability is often subjective without physical laxity of the joint and is a result of deficits in proprioception, postural control, or muscle strength.[3] Mechanical lateral ankle instability results as a structural deficiency in the surrounding ligaments of the ankle leading to increased laxity and unnecessary motion about the joint.[3] Both mechanical and functional ankle instability, if improperly managed, can put athletes at risk of further injury. Injury to the syndesmosis, sometimes referred to as high ankle sprain, is an additional form of ankle instability that is often more severe in extent and outcome.[5] Disruption of the anatomic structures of the syndesmosis can also lead to mechanical ankle instability, pain, and delayed recovery.

With the frequency of ankle sprains, lateral ligament instability, and syndesmotic injuries, it is essential to understand the underlying cause and risk factors for these conditions. Greater understanding allows for proper prevention, diagnoses, and treatment of athletes with these conditions. Appropriate initial treatment is critical to returning athletes to sport and preventing long-term morbidity. This article investigates the epidemiology, anatomy, diagnosis, and management of patients with ankles sprains and lateral ankle injuries.

EPIDEMIOLOGY AND RISK FACTORS

The incidence rate of ankle sprains is 2.15 per 1000 person-years in the general population of the United States.[6] However, incidence rates increase with exposure to sport occurring at a rate of 3.4 injuries per 1000 athlete exposures in the National Basketball Association and 2.06 per 1000 athlete-hours in soccer players.[7,8] Similarly, lateral ankle sprain and syndesmotic sprain are the most common foot and ankle injuries in collegiate football players occurring in 31% and 15% of players, respectively.[9] Although ankle injury is more common in collision sports, ankle sprains are frequently reported as the most common injury regardless of the type of athletic exposure.[7-12]

The incidence of ankle sprains also varies with demographics. Ankle sprains are more common in younger age groups, 15 to 19 years of age, and specifically males.[6] Some studies have shown an increased incidence in female athletes, whereas others demonstrate increased incidence in males.[6,13] The true difference in gender may be sport specific. Several studies have shown increased frequency of ankle sprains in female basketball players compared with their male counterparts or when compared with their female colleagues who participate in other sports, such as lacrosse, field hockey, volleyball, and soccer.[14-16]

Multiple studies have attempted to identify specific anatomic and physical risk factors for ankles sprains and chronic ankle instability. There is evidence to suggest increased frequency of ankle sprains in athletes with increasing body mass index and lower physical activity.[17,18] Some authors suggest athletes with muscle imbalances have an increased risk for ankle instability, whereas others have found significant risk with how the calcaneus moves during gait.[17,18] Poor postural stability has also been identified as a possible risk factor.[19]

Previous authors support the theory that some of these risks can be modified, whereas others are fundamental to the athlete and cannot be changed. Modifiable risk factors for ankle sprains include body mass index; use of preventative therapies, such as braces or tape; strengthening; participation in sport; player positions; and even playing surfaces and equipment.[9,13,20,21] Nonmodifiable risk factors include demographic factors, such as age, gender, and race, and anatomic factors, such as limb alignment, anatomic variation, and joint laxity.[13,18,19] However, the true relevance of these risk factors, modifiable or not, are difficult to discern because large systematic reviews evaluating such factors have poor consensus.[22,23]

Identifying risk factors and demographic contributions for syndesmosis injury in athletes has been more difficult with limited studies showing significance for specific risk factors. However, vertical jump distance and balance may play a role.[12] Additionally, in football, player position has been shown to have different rates of ankle injury.[9]

PATHOANATOMY

Unlike other joints in the body the tibiotalar joint is inherently stable given the complementing structures of the medial malleolus of the tibia and the medial shoulder of the talus. This structural stability continues on the lateral side with lateral malleolus of the fibula; however, the fibula is able to change positions to accommodate motion of the talus during ankle movement.[24] The boney constraints of the medial and lateral aspects of the ankle joint provide significant stability in the coronal plane attributing to the predominant motion of the tibiotalar joint being plantar and dorsiflexion in the sagittal plane.

The relationship of the fibula to the tibia is maintained by the ligamentous structures of the syndesmosis. These ligamentous structures include the anterior inferior tibiofibular ligament, posterior inferior tibiofibular ligament, inferior transverse ligament, interosseous ligament, and interosseous membrane. These structures allow for an increase in the intermalleolar distance during the swing phase of gait to accommodate for the dorsiflexion and clearance of the foot, and the distance decreases during the stance phase to provide stability to the ankle joint.[24] Recurrent injury to the syndesmosis in professional athletes has been reported to result in tibiofibular synostosis and/or heterotopic ossification leading to pain with impact activities and restricted range of motion.[12,24]

The surrounding ligamentous support of the ankle joint is also crucial to adding stability to the joint. The anterior talofibular ligament (ATFL) prevents anterior translation of the talus relative to the tibia and is often the first structure injured during an ankle sprain.[25] The calcaneofibular ligament (CFL) resists inversion of talus relative to the tibia but also provides stability to the subtalar joint; it is the second structure injured during an ankle sprain.[25] The posterior talofibular ligament prevents posterior translation of the talus relative to the tibia when the ankle is in neutral plantar flexion, but is rarely injured during inversion injury to the ankle.[26]

The superior aspect of the anterior lateral joint capsule is often overlooked as a structure that provides stability to the ankle. However, cadaveric studies have demonstrated that disruption of the anterior lateral joint capsule results in 18% of joint displacement in grade I ankle sprains and up to 33% of displacement in grade III injuries.[25] Similarly, the stabilization provided by the capsule is even more critical in chronic lateral ligament laxity.[27]

The musculature surrounding the ankle joint provides active stability to the ankle joint during motion. Specifically peroneus longus and brevis assist with counteracting inversion forces during injury. Injury to the peroneal tendons in patients with chronic ankle instability is thought to be the result of repetitive compression of the tendons along the posterior aspect of the fibula.[28] In addition, there is a risk of tendon subluxation given the orientation of fibers of the CFL and superior peroneal retinaculum.

The histology of acutely injured lateral ankle ligaments is not unlike other areas of anatomy. Broström and Sundelin[27] reported a predominance of hemorrhage and fibrous exudate exists immediately following injury, which is replaced by granulocytic infiltration, mononuclear cells, and fibroblast a few days following injury. Chronically lax ligaments, even though previously injured, are able to remodel into parallel collagen bundles not unlike normal ligamentous structure.[27] This is in contrast to the degeneration that occurs in chronically injured tendons, such as the Achilles.

PATIENT EVALUATION

Critical to the treatment of ankle sprains and lateral ankle instability is patient evaluation through history and physical examination. Patients often present with difficulty weight bearing, lateral ankle pain, swelling, and ecchymosis.[29] Clinicians should differentiate a first-time ankle sprain from recurrent injury and discuss the mechanism of injury. Patients often report the sensation of their ankle giving way or describe multiple episodes of instability.[3] Symptoms of instability should also be discussed to determine functional from mechanical instability because treatment varies.[3] Patient level of function and athletic participation may also affect treatment and rehabilitation.

The physical examination is fundamental in the evaluation of patients with ankle sprains and lateral ankle instability. As with any patient with foot or ankle symptoms, evaluation of the hind foot alignment for planovalgus or cavovarus deformity should not be overlooked. Patients with a cavus deformity are more likely to develop attenuated lateral ligaments and subsequent lateral ankle instability.[30] These patients should be addressed with caution because the underlying cause of the ankle problem is likely from their malalignment and traditional soft tissue reconstruction options are likely to fail. The ability to weight bear following injury and the specific anatomic location of pain on examination can assist with determining the need for imaging using the Ottawa ankle rules.[29] Range of motion and gait are used to discern the acuity and severity of the injury at the time of evaluation.

Provocative tests for determining functional from mechanical instability include talar tilt, anterior drawer, squeeze, and external rotation stress tests. These tests may be less useful in the acute setting because of guarding on the patient's part. Talar tilt evaluates the integrity of the CFL and is performed with inversion stress to the lateral ankle.[1] Anterior drawer evaluates ATFL and is performed by directing and anterior force to the talus while stabilizing the tibia.[31] It is likely to be positive in patients with chronic injury as evident by the suction sign.[1,2] Anterior lateral drawer test is performed similarly to the traditional test only it allows for rotation of the talus about the intact medial ankle ligaments. It may identify the more subtle injury to the ATFL because detection of incompetence of that structure is not limited by the deltoid.[31] Squeeze test is used if there is suspicion for a syndesmotic injury; patients report ankle pain with squeezing of the fibula against the tibia at the mid-calf level.[5] External rotation stress test also evaluates the syndesmosis; the proximal tibia is stabilized and an external rotational force is applied to the foot and is considered positive if patients complain of pain.[1,5]

IMAGING

Should history and physical examination prompt further evaluation with imaging, clinicians should start with weight bearing standard three-view radiographs of the ankle and foot.[29] Additional anteroposterior and lateral radiographs of the leg are also critical to rule out syndesmotic injury or a high fibula fracture.[5] Although most patients with ankle sprains are likely to have normal radiographs, they should be used to rule out fracture or dislocation in the acute setting, and a tarsal coalition often associated with recurrent ankle sprains.[29,32] Stress radiographs or fluoroscopic imaging evaluating talar tilt and anterior talar translation can help evaluate the integrity of the lateral ankle ligaments. According to Lee and colleagues,[33] disruption of the posterior talo-fibular ligament is likely to be the only significant variable contributing to anterior talar translation; talar tilt on stress radiographs is affected by not only the integrity to the ATFL but also age and gender of the patient. Given the variability of stress views to the degree of ligamentous injury many authors question their clinical utility. However, knowledge of the extent of the lateral ankle instability on preoperative radiographs (particularly when asymmetric) provides assistance with anatomic reconstruction via intraoperative radiographic evaluation and can assist with radiographic evaluation postoperatively.[34]

Because radiographs are often of minimal benefit in patients with lateral ankle insta-bility, MRI is frequently prescribed. MRI should be reserved for patients with chronic lateral ankle instability who fail a course of initial conservative treatment or who have unexplained pain in association with the ligament disorder. Although MRI of the ankle has excellent intraobserver reliability and positive predictive value for injury to the ATLF, its sensitivity is low for imaging, between 76% and 84%.[35] These limita-tions continue when evaluating for concomitant injuries of the ankle. Although MRI may identify associated pathology, such as osteochondral lesions, peroneal tendon tears, and loose bodies, the sensitivity of identifying such is still lower than with arthroscopy.[36,37] Clinicians should be systematic in evaluating the ankle joint during arthroscopy so as not to overlook these subtle concomitant injuries.

Ultrasound has recently become more widely used in the evaluation of musculoskel-etal injuries. This modality can demonstrate increased elongation of the ATFL with an anterior drawer applied.[38] Similarly, syndesmotic injuries can also be evaluated with ultrasound techniques. Injury of the interosseous membrane is suspected if there is disruption of the normal linear hyperechoic structure between the tibia and fibula.[5] Un-fortunately, ultrasound remains operator dependent with difficulty in reproducibility and interpretation.

PREVENTATIVE TREATMENT

Preventative treatment of ankle sprains and subsequent lateral ankle instability begins with identifying modifiable risk factors. Deficiencies in balance are addressed with sin-gle limb balance training and neuromuscluar control.[39,40] This training seems to be most useful at decreasing rates of ankle injury in patients that are at increased risk of injury, such as those with increased body mass index or those with history of pre-vious injury.[39,40] Addressing deficiencies in ankle range of motion and muscle strength of the lower extremity has lower levels of evidence for injury prevention, but can easily be added to an athlete's training.[39]

Some authors have advocated the use of bracing to prevent ankle sprains. These braces provide additional lateral and medial mechanical support.[15] Although bracing had been shown to be useful in selective sports it is probably most useful in patients with recurrent ankle sprains rather than prophylaxis.[10,39]

Similar to bracing is the practice of taping. Taping is thought to assist the athlete by making up for the deficit in proprioception following the initial ankle injury. Although experimental models have difficulty validating this theory,[41] taping has proved to be effective in decreasing ankle injury in patients with previous injury and should be considered as preventative treatment.[10,39]

NONPHARMACOLOGIC TREATMENT

First time ankle sprains should be treated similarly to other musculoskeletal injuries us-ing the PRICE acronym: protection, rest, ice, compression, and elevation.[39] Following improvement of initial symptoms, patients should progress to weight bearing as tolerated. Early range of motion has been shown to have improved functional outcomes and has equal pain scores compared with those treated with prolonged periods of immobilization.[42,43] An elastic compression wrap with an air stirrup type of brace can allow for a return to baseline walking speed faster than treatment with a brace or wrap alone.[44] Patients with low-grade syndesmotic injuries should be immobilized and institute protected weight bearing for a longer period of time, perhaps 3 to 4 weeks, as compared with athletes with a simple low-grade inversion ankle sprain.[45]

Physical therapy and rehabilitation are critical in preventing functional instability and decreasing a patient's risk for recurrent injury. Supervised physical therapy has better outcomes with regard to strength and proprioception for ankle sprains in the short term; however, improvement in reinjury rates and long-term functional results are similar to home therapy plans.[46] Consideration should be given to an evaluation with MRI for those patients with protracted functional instability or pain.

PHARMACOLOGIC TREATMENT OPTIONS

In addition to nonpharmacologic treatment, pharmacologic treatment assists with pain control, inflammation, and swelling. These medications should be used in conjunction with nonpharmacologic treatments. Nonsteroidal anti-inflammatory drugs in the form of cyclooxygenase inhibitors or specific cyclooxygenase-2 inhibitors, such as celecoxib are more effective than placebo at treating pain in patients with lateral ankle sprain.[47] Topical nonsteroidal anti-inflammatory drugs, such as diclofenac diethylamine 2.32% gel, have also been shown to be safe and effective for ankle sprains.[48] Acetaminophen extended release is as useful as ibuprofen with minimal side effects.[49] New treatments with platelet-rich plasma injections have shown minimal improvement in randomized studies and are likely of limited use in lateral ankle sprains.[50]

SURGICAL TREATMENT

An acute ankle sprain is not a typical indication for surgical intervention because immediate reconstruction or repair of the lateral ligaments has not shown to provide any improvement in long-term functional outcomes.[51] On the contrary, those patients that develop chronic instability are unlikely to have improvement in their symptoms without surgical intervention.[4] The increased risk for developing posttraumatic arthritis in these patients is suggested but remains in question.[4] It is our belief that patients who have failed formal rehabilitation of prior ankle sprains and have evidence for mechanical instability benefit from lateral ligament reconstruction.

Surgical treatment of lateral ankle instability varies depending on the specific type of lateral ligament reconstruction. The goal is to provide a stable ankle no matter what procedure is performed. Broström[2] described his technique for direct repair of the lateral ankle ligaments (ATFL only) with suture in 1966. Gould augmented this technique in 1980 with advancement of the extensor retinaculum and the procedure has been further modified by repairing both the ATFL and CFL back to the fibula using bone tunnels or suture anchors.[52,53] The modified Broström-Gould procedure provides an anatomic reconstruction of the lateral ligaments and is the most widely used.

The Broström-Gould techniques may fail to provide adequate stability in those patients found to have poor soft tissue envelope because of chronic injury or underlying cavovarus. Therefore additional reconstruction techniques have been described and often use modifications of the local anatomy to provide stability (**Fig. 1**). For example, Evans[54] described in 1953 a transposition of the peroneus brevis tendon through a

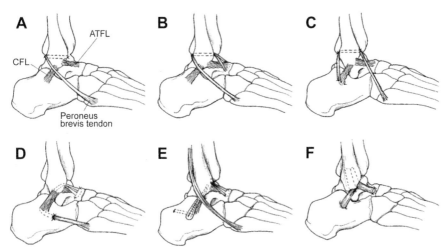

Fig. 1. Augmented reconstructions. (*A*) The Evans reconstruction uses a tenodesis of the peroneus brevis tendon to the fibula. (*B*) The Watson-Jones procedure reconstructs the ATFL in addition to tenodesis of the peroneus brevis tendon. (*C*) The Chrisman-Snook procedure uses a split peroneus brevis tendon to reconstruct the ATFL and CFL. (*D*) The procedure developed by Colville also uses a split peroneus brevis tendon to reconstruct the ATFL and CFL in an anatomic fashion without limiting subtalar motion. (*E*) The Anderson procedure uses the plantaris tendon to anatomically reconstruct both lateral ligaments without limiting subtalar motion. (*F*) The Sjølin technique uses periosteal flaps to augment an anatomic repair. (*From* Colville MR. Surgical treatment of the unstable ankle. J Am Acad Orthop Surg 1998;6:374; with permission.)

bone tunnel in the distal fibula followed by reattachment of the tendon to its remaining distal portion. Today this procedure is more commonly done, as described by Girard and colleagues,[55] using an anterior slip of the peroneus brevis as a checkrein, therefore avoiding complete disruption of the tendon and preserving most tendon function (**Fig. 2**). Similarly, the original Chrisman-Snook procedure or its modifications use an anterior slip of the peroneus brevis or allograft tendon grafts. In addition to rerouting

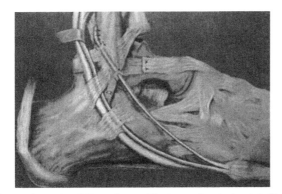

Fig. 2. The end-to-end repair of the calcaneofibular and anterior talofibular ligaments is achieved with nonabsorbable suture. The split tendon is rerouted through a drill hole in the distal fibula and is secured at both ends. (*From* Girard P, Anderson RB, Davis WH, et al. Clinical evaluation of the modified Broström-Evans procedure to restore ankle stability. Foot Ankle Int 1999;20(4):246–52.)

the tendon through the distal fibula, it is routed through a second bone tunnel in the calcaneus to recreate the CFL. In the original description the tendon is further sutured back to itself near the anterolateral ankle.[56]

There are several other procedures described to address lateral ankle instability. Given the dynamic stability the peroneal tendons provide, there is a theoretical reason to avoid violating them during reconstruction. As such, authors have described using extensor tendon from the fourth toe or semitendinosus allograft.[57,58] As an option to soft tissue augmentation the repair can also use suture tape with reported good results.[59] Patients who have lateral ankle instability in the setting of moderate-severe varus malalignment may benefit from supramalleolar or lateralizing calcaneal osteotomies, in addition to a more robust and augmented soft tissue reconstruction.[60]

Unstable syndesmotic injuries have traditionally been treated with rigid internal stabilization to achieve and maintain anatomic alignment, thus allowing for proper healing while preventing further injury. There has been controversy surrounding the type, size, and extent of screw fixation. Cadaveric studies have failed to show any significant difference between 3.5-mm and 4.5-mm screws or quadricortical versus tricortical fixation.[61] Furthermore, the syndesmosis is a true and functional joint, with inherent motion occurring between the fibula and tibia. As a result, implant removal has been advocated before returning the athlete to full activity to avoid the potential complications of screw breakage.[45] However, more recent clinical data refute this assumption, showing no correlation between screw breakage and pain.[62] To avoid this situation and to provide more physiologic, flexible fixation, there is a recent trend to treat these injuries with a modified suture button construct. Studies have shown little difference between modified suture construct for syndesmotic fixation versus screw fixation in a cadaveric model.[63] However, location of the fixation does seem to be important because there is increased displacement if fixation is placed too close to the tibial plafond.[64]

SURGICAL OUTCOMES, REHABILITATION, AND RETURN TO PLAY

Surgical outcomes for lateral ligament reconstruction are favorable. Maffulli and colleagues[65] published long-term results on athletes following a Broström procedure and found 58% were able to return to their preinjury level of sport, 16% were still competing but at a lower level, and 26% had discontinued sport participation but were still physically active. Similarly, long-term results of arthroscopic-assisted Broström-Gould are also positive. In Nery and colleagues's[66] cohort of 38 patients, only two patients had low functional scores. There was no difference in functional score between patients that had microfracture for osteochondral lesions at the time of surgery and those who had lateral ligament reconstruction alone after a follow-up of 9.8 years.

Return to play following syndesmosis ankle injury is often longer and of greater variability compared with lateral ankle sprains.[5] However, the outcome for patients undergoing treatment with greater than 1 year of syndesmotic instability are promising. Ryan and Rodriguez[67] showed that at 2 years follow-up 11 of 14 patients were able to return to their preinjury level of competition after treatment with arthroscopic debridement of the syndesmosis and fixation. As expected, the more severe the syndesmotic injury, the longer a player is unable to play. Miller and colleagues[5] found a positive correlation between the height of the syndesmotic injury and the number of days to return to play with the average time out of football being 15.5 days.

COMPLICATIONS

Although serious complications for lateral ligament reconstructions are rare, no surgery is without risk. Complications include infection, osteoarthritis, neuroma, disathesias, and recurrence of instabilty.[2] Complications for operatively treated syndesmosis injuries are similar to lateral ligament reconstruction. However, unique to syndesmotic operative treatment is obtaining an accurate reduction of the joint, which is difficult to evaluate intraoperatively, especially with fluoroscopy.[68] As a result, malreduction of the syndesmosis has been reported in up to 52% of cases. Even evaluation of the reduction on computed tomography can be inconsistent depending on the method of measurements used.[68,69] In the end, the morbidity of having a malreduced syndesmosis is questioned because implants are routinely removed or break allowing the fibula to return to its original anatomic location.

SUMMARY

Ankle sprains are an exceedingly common injury in an athletic population. Modifiable risk factors for injury need to be identified and addressed before engaging in athletic activity. Acute ankle injury treatment includes activity modification and pain control with focus on returning to weight bearing and range of motion when symptoms allow. Physical therapy focusing on strengthening and proprioception is the mainstay of recovery. When patients return to baseline, it is recommended that they return to the athletic field with external support in the form of a brace or tape apparatus to prevent further injury. Athletes with dysfunction that fail to respond to physical therapy or have recurrent injuries are indicated for lateral ligament reconstruction.

REFERENCES

1. Coughlin MJ, Saltzman CL, Anderson RB. Mann's surgery of the foot and ankle, 2-volume set: expert consult: online and print, 9e (Coughlin, surgery of the foot and ankle 2v set). Philadelphia: Saunders Elsevier Inc; 2013. p. 2336.
2. Broström L. Sprained ankles. VI. Surgical treatment of "chronic" ligament ruptures. Acta Chir Scand 1966;132(5):551–65.
3. Chen H, Li HY, Zhang J, et al. Difference in postural control between patients with functional and mechanical ankle instability. Foot Ankle Int 2014;35(10):1068–74.
4. Löfvenberg R, Kärrholm J, Lund B. The outcome of nonoperated patients with chronic lateral instability of the ankle: a 20-year follow-up study. Foot Ankle Int 1994;15(4):165–9.
5. Miller BS, Downie BK, Johnson PD, et al. Time to return to play after high ankle sprains in collegiate football players: a prediction model. Sports Health 2012; 4(6):504–9.
6. Waterman BR, Owens BD, Davey S, et al. The epidemiology of ankle sprains in the United States. J Bone Joint Surg Am 2010;92(13):2279–84.
7. Drakos MC, Domb B, Starkey C, et al. Injury in the National Basketball Association: a 17-year overview. Sports Health 2010;2(4):284–90.
8. Kofotolis ND, Kellis E, Vlachopoulos SP. Ankle sprain injuries and risk factors in amateur soccer players during a 2-year period. Am J Sports Med 2007;35(3): 458–66.
9. Kaplan LD, Jost PW, Honkamp N, et al. Incidence and variance of foot and ankle injuries in elite college football players. Am J Orthop (Belle Mead NJ) 2011;40(1): 40–4.
10. Dizon JM, Reyes JJ. A systematic review on the effectiveness of external ankle supports in the prevention of inversion ankle sprains among elite and recreational players. J Sci Med Sport 2010;13(3):309–17.
11. Sankey RA, Brooks JH, Kemp SP, et al. The epidemiology of ankle injuries in professional rugby union players. Am J Sports Med 2008;36(12):2415–24.

12. Sman AD, Hiller CE, Rae K, et al. Predictive factors for ankle syndesmosis injury in football players: a prospective study. J Sci Med Sport 2014;17(6):586–90.

13. McCriskin BJ, Cameron KL, Orr JD, et al. Management and prevention of acute and chronic lateral ankle instability in athletic patient populations. World J Orthop 2015;6(2):161–71.

14. Beynnon BD, Vacek PM, Murphy D, et al. First-time inversion ankle ligament trauma: the effects of sex, level of competition, and sport on the incidence of injury. Am J Sports Med 2005;33(10):1485–91.

15. Frey C, Feder KS, Sleight J. Prophylactic ankle brace use in high school volleyball players: a prospective study. Foot Ankle Int 2010;31(4):296–300.

16. Hosea TM, Carey CC, Harrer MF. The gender issue: epidemiology of ankle injuries in athletes who participate in basketball. Clin Orthop Relat Res 2000;372: 45–9.

17. Fousekis K, Tsepis E, Vagenas G. Intrinsic risk factors of noncontact ankle sprains in soccer: a prospective study on 100 professional players. Am J Sports Med 2012;40(8):1842–50.

18. Willems TM, Witvrouw E, Delbaere K, et al. Intrinsic risk factors for inversion ankle sprains in male subjects: a prospective study. Am J Sports Med 2005;33(3): 415–23.

19. Willems TM, Witvrouw E, Delbaere K, et al. Intrinsic risk factors for inversion ankle sprains in females: a prospective study. Scand J Med Sci Sports 2005;15(5): 336–45.

20. Hershman EB, Anderson R, Bergfeld JA, et al. An analysis of specific lower extremity injury rates on grass and FieldTurf playing surfaces in National Football League Games: 2000-2009 seasons. Am J Sports Med 2012;40(10):2200–5.

21. Janda DH, Bir C, Kedroske B. A comparison of standard vs. breakaway bases: an analysis of a preventative intervention for softball and baseball foot and ankle injuries. Foot Ankle Int 2001;22(10):810–6.

22. Hiller CE, Nightingale EJ, Lin CW, et al. Characteristics of people with recurrent ankle sprains: a systematic review with meta-analysis. Br J Sports Med 2011; 45(8):660–72.

23. Witchalls J, Blanch P, Waddington G, et al. Intrinsic functional deficits associated with increased risk of ankle injuries: a systematic review with meta-analysis. Br J Sports Med 2012;46(7):515–23.

24. Whiteside LA, Reynolds FC, Ellsasser JC. Tibiofibular synostosis and recurrent ankle sprains in high performance athletes. Am J Sports Med 1978;6(4):204–8.

25. Boardman DL, Liu SH. Contribution of the anterolateral joint capsule to the mechanical stability of the ankle. Clin Orthop Relat Res 1997;341:224–32.

26. Clanton TO, Campbell KJ, Wilson KJ, et al. Qualitative and quantitative anatomic investigation of the lateral ankle ligaments for surgical reconstruction procedures. J Bone Joint Surg Am 2014;96(12):e98.

27. Broström L, Sundelin P. Sprained ankles. IV. Histologic changes in recent and "chronic" ligament ruptures. Acta Chir Scand 1966;132(3):248–53.

28. Bonnin M, Tavernier T, Bouysset M. Split lesions of the peroneus brevis tendon in chronic ankle laxity. Am J Sports Med 1997;25(5):699–703.

29. Bachmann LM, Kolb E, Koller MT, et al. Accuracy of Ottawa ankle rules to exclude fractures of the ankle and mid-foot: systematic review. BMJ 2003;326(7386):417.

30. Larsen E, Angermann P. Association of ankle instability and foot deformity. Acta Orthop Scand 1990;61(2):136–9.

31. Miller AG, Myers SH, Parks BG, et al. Anterolateral drawer versus anterior drawer test for ankle instability: a biomechanical model. Foot Ankle Int 2016;37(4): 407–10.

32. Omey ML, Micheli LJ. Foot and ankle problems in the young athlete. Med Sci Sports Exerc 1999;31(7 Suppl):S470–86.

33. Lee KM, Chung CY, Kwon SS, et al. Relationship between stress ankle radiographs and injured ligaments on MRI. Skeletal Radiol 2013;42(11):1537–42.

34. Haytmanek CT, Williams BT, James EW, et al. Radiographic identification of the primary lateral ankle structures. Am J Sports Med 2015;43(1):79–87.

35. Kim YS, Kim YB, Kim TG, et al. Reliability and validity of magnetic resonance imaging for the evaluation of the anterior talofibular ligament in patients undergoing ankle arthroscopy. Arthroscopy 2015;31(8):1540–7.

36. O'Neill PJ, Van Aman SE, Guyton GP. Is MRI adequate to detect lesions in patients with ankle instability. Clin Orthop Relat Res 2010;468(4):1115–9.

37. Roemer FW, Jomaah N, Niu J, et al. Ligamentous injuries and the risk of associated tissue damage in acute ankle sprains in athletes: a cross-sectional MRI Study. Am J Sports Med 2014;42(7):1549–57.

38. Croy T, Saliba SA, Saliba E, et al. Differences in lateral ankle laxity measured via stress ultrasonography in individuals with chronic ankle instability, ankle sprain copers, and healthy individuals. J Orthop Sports Phys Ther 2012;42(7):593–600.

39. Kaminski TW, Hertel J, Amendola N, et al. National Athletic Trainers' Association position statement: conservative management and prevention of ankle sprains in athletes. J Athl Train 2013;48(4):528–45.

40. McHugh MP, Tyler TF, Mirabella MR, et al. The effectiveness of a balance training intervention in reducing the incidence of noncontact ankle sprains in high school football players. Am J Sports Med 2007;35(8):1289–94.

41. Refshauge KM, Raymond J, Kilbreath SL, et al. The effect of ankle taping on detection of inversion-eversion movements in participants with recurrent ankle sprain. Am J Sports Med 2009;37(2):371–5.

42. Bleakley CM, O'Connor SR, Tully MA, et al. Effect of accelerated rehabilitation on function after ankle sprain: randomised controlled trial. BMJ 2010;340:c1964.

43. Prado MP, Mendes AA, Amodio DT, et al. A comparative, prospective, and randomized study of two conservative treatment protocols for first-episode lateral ankle ligament injuries. Foot Ankle Int 2014;35(3):201–6.

44. Beynnon BD, Renström PA, Haugh L, et al. A prospective, randomized clinical investigation of the treatment of first-time ankle sprains. Am J Sports Med 2006;34(9):1401–12.

45. Miller TL, Skalak T. Evaluation and treatment recommendations for acute injuries to the ankle syndesmosis without associated fracture. Sports Med 2014;44(2): 179–88.

46. Feger MA, Herb CC, Fraser JJ, et al. Supervised rehabilitation versus home exercise in the treatment of acute ankle sprains: a systematic review. Clin Sports Med 2015;34(2):329–46.

47. Ekman EF, Fiechtner JJ, Levy S, et al. Efficacy of celecoxib versus ibuprofen in the treatment of acute pain: a multicenter, double-blind, randomized controlled trial in acute ankle sprain. Am J Orthop (Belle Mead NJ) 2002;31(8):445–51.

48. Predel HG, Hamelsky S, Gold M, et al. Efficacy and safety of diclofenac diethylamine 2.32% gel in acute ankle sprain. Med Sci Sports Exerc 2012;44(9): 1629–36.

49. Dalton JD, Schweinle JE. Randomized controlled noninferiority trial to compare extended release acetaminophen and ibuprofen for the treatment of ankle sprains. Ann Emerg Med 2006;48(5):615–23.
50. Rowden A, Dominici P, D'Orazio J, et al. Double-blind, randomized, placebo-controlled study evaluating the use of platelet-rich plasma therapy (PRP) for acute ankle sprains in the emergency department. J Emerg Med 2015;49(4): 546–51.
51. Kaikkonen A, Kannus P, Järvinen M. Surgery versus functional treatment in ankle ligament tears. A prospective study. Clin Orthop Relat Res 1996;326:194–202.
52. Gould N, Seligson D, Gassman J. Early and late repair of lateral ligament of the ankle. Foot Ankle 1980;1(2):84–9.
53. Hu CY, Lee KB, Song EK, et al. Comparison of bone tunnel and suture anchor techniques in the modified Broström procedure for chronic lateral ankle instability. Am J Sports Med 2013;41(8):1877–84.
54. Evans DL. Recurrent instability of the ankle; a method of surgical treatment. Proc R Soc Med 1953;46(5):343–4.
55. Girard P, Anderson RB, Davis WH, et al. Clinical evaluation of the modified Brostrom-Evans procedure to restore ankle stability. Foot Ankle Int 1999;20(4): 246–52.
56. Chrisman OD, Snook GA. Reconstruction of lateral ligament tears of the ankle. An experimental study and clinical evaluation of seven patients treated by a new modification of the Elmslie procedure. J Bone Joint Surg Am 1969;51(5):904–12.
57. Ahn JH, Choy WS, Kim HY. Reconstruction of the lateral ankle ligament with a long extensor tendon graft of the fourth toe. Am J Sports Med 2011;39(3):637–44.
58. Clanton TO, Viens NA, Campbell KJ, et al. Anterior talofibular ligament ruptures, part 2: biomechanical comparison of anterior talofibular ligament reconstruction using semitendinosus allografts with the intact ligament. Am J Sports Med 2014;42(2):412–6.
59. Cho BK, Park KJ, Kim SW, et al. Minimal invasive suture-tape augmentation for chronic ankle instability. Foot Ankle Int 2015;36(11):1330–8.
60. Mann HA, Filippi J, Myerson MS. Intra-articular opening medial tibial wedge osteotomy (plafond-plasty) for the treatment of intra-articular varus ankle arthritis and instability. Foot Ankle Int 2012;33(4):255–61.
61. Markolf KL, Jackson SR, McAllister DR. Syndesmosis fixation using dual 3.5 mm and 4.5 mm screws with tricortical and quadricortical purchase: a biomechanical study. Foot Ankle Int 2013;34(5):734–9.
62. Hamid N, Loeffler BJ, Braddy W, et al. Outcome after fixation of ankle fractures with an injury to the syndesmosis: the effect of the syndesmosis screw. J Bone Joint Surg Br 2009;91(8):1069–73.
63. Ebramzadeh E, Knutsen AR, Sangiorgio SN, et al. Biomechanical comparison of syndesmotic injury fixation methods using a cadaveric model. Foot Ankle Int 2013;34(12):1710–7.
64. Miller RS, Weinhold PS, Dahners LE. Comparison of tricortical screw fixation versus a modified suture construct for fixation of ankle syndesmosis injury: a biomechanical study. J Orthop Trauma 1999;13(1):39–42.
65. Maffulli N, Del Buono A, Maffulli GD, et al. Isolated anterior talofibular ligament Broström repair for chronic lateral ankle instability: 9-year follow-up. Am J Sports Med 2013;41(4):858–64.
66. Nery C, Raduan F, Del Buono A, et al. Arthroscopic-assisted Broström-Gould for chronic ankle instability: a long-term follow-up. Am J Sports Med 2011;39(11): 2381–8.

67. Ryan PM, Rodriguez RM. Outcomes and return to activity after operative repair of chronic latent syndesmotic instability. Foot Ankle Int 2016;37(2):192–7.
68. Koenig SJ, Tornetta P, Merlin G, et al. Can we tell if the syndesmosis is reduced using fluoroscopy. J Orthop Trauma 2015;29(9):e326–30.
69. Knops SP, Kohn MA, Hansen EN, et al. Rotational malreduction of the syndesmosis: reliability and accuracy of computed tomography measurement methods. Foot Ankle Int 2013;34(10):1403–10.

Index

Note: Page numbers of article titles are in **boldface** type.

Clin Sports Med 35 (2016) 711–716
http://dx.doi.org/10.1016/S0278-5919(16)30060-6
0278-5919/16/$ – see front matter

sportsmed.theclinics.com

UNITED STATES POSTAL SERVICE

Statement of Ownership, Management, and Circulation
(All Periodicals Publications Except Requester Publications)

1. Publication Title	2. Publication Number		3. Filing Date
CLINICS IN SPORTS MEDICINE	000 – 702		9/18/2016

4. Issue Frequency	5. Number of Issues Published Annually	6. Annual Subscription Price
JAN, APR, JUL, OCT	4	$324.00

7. Complete Mailing Address of Known Office of Publication (Not printer) (Street, city, county, state, and ZIP+4®)	Contact Person
ELSEVIER INC. 360 PARK AVENUE SOUTH NEW YORK, NY 10010-1710	STEPHEN R. BUSHING
	Telephone (Include area code) 215-239-3688

8. Complete Mailing Address of Headquarters or General Business Office of Publisher (Not printer)

ELSEVIER INC.
360 PARK AVENUE SOUTH
NEW YORK, NY 10010-1710

9. Full Names and Complete Mailing Addresses of Publisher, Editor, and Managing Editor (Do not leave blank)

Publisher (Name and complete mailing address)

LINDA BELFUS, ELSEVIER INC.
1600 JOHN F KENNEDY BLVD. SUITE 1800
PHILADELPHIA, PA 19103-2899

Editor (Name and complete mailing address)

JENNIFER FLYNN-BRIGGS, ELSEVIER INC.
1600 JOHN F KENNEDY BLVD. SUITE 1800
PHILADELPHIA, PA 19103-2899

Managing Editor (Name and complete mailing address)

ADRIANNE BRIGIDO, ELSEVIER INC.
1600 JOHN F KENNEDY BLVD. SUITE 1800
PHILADELPHIA, PA 19103-2899

10. Owner (Do not leave blank. If the publication is owned by a corporation, give the name and address of the corporation immediately followed by the names and addresses of all stockholders owning or holding 1 percent or more of the total amount of stock. If not owned by a corporation, give the names and addresses of the individual owners. If owned by a partnership or other unincorporated firm, give its name and address as well as those of each individual owner. If the publication is published by a nonprofit organization, give its name and address.)

Full Name	Complete Mailing Address
WHOLLY OWNED SUBSIDIARY OF REED/ELSEVIER, US HOLDINGS	1600 JOHN F KENNEDY BLVD. SUITE 1800 PHILADELPHIA, PA 19103-2899

11. Known Bondholders, Mortgagees, and Other Security Holders Owning or Holding 1 Percent or More of Total Amount of Bonds, Mortgages, or Other Securities. If none, check box. ▶ ☐ None

Full Name	Complete Mailing Address
N/A	

12. Tax Status (For completion by nonprofit organizations authorized to mail at nonprofit rates) (Check one)
The purpose, function, and nonprofit status of this organization and the exempt status for federal income tax purposes:
☐ Has Not Changed During Preceding 12 Months
☐ Has Changed During Preceding 12 Months (Publisher must submit explanation of change with this statement)

13. Publication Title	14. Issue Date for Circulation Data Below
CLINICS IN SPORTS MEDICINE	JULY 2016

15. Extent and Nature of Circulation			Average No. Copies Each Issue During Preceding 12 Months	No. Copies of Single Issue Published Nearest to Filing Date
a. Total Number of Copies (Net press run)			463	508
b. Paid Circulation (By Mail and Outside the Mail)	(1)	Mailed Outside-County Paid Subscriptions Stated on PS Form 3541 (Include paid distribution above nominal rate, advertiser's proof copies, and exchange copies)	228	211
	(2)	Mailed In-County Paid Subscriptions Stated on PS Form 3541 (Include paid distribution above nominal rate, advertiser's proof copies, and exchange copies)	0	0
	(3)	Paid Distribution Outside the Mails Including Sales Through Dealers and Carriers, Street Vendors, Counter Sales, and Other Paid Distribution Outside USPS®	76	76
	(4)	Paid Distribution by Other Classes of Mail Through the USPS (e.g., First-Class Mail®)	0	0
c. Total Paid Distribution (Sum of 15b (1), (2), (3), and (4))		▶	304	287
d. Free or Nominal Rate Distribution (By Mail and Outside the Mail)	(1)	Free or Nominal Rate Outside-County Copies included on PS Form 3541	52	48
	(2)	Free or Nominal Rate In-County Copies Included on PS Form 3541	0	0
	(3)	Free or Nominal Rate Copies Mailed at Other Classes Through the USPS (e.g., First-Class Mail)	0	0
	(4)	Free or Nominal Rate Distribution Outside the Mail (Carriers or other means)	18	23
e. Total Free or Nominal Rate Distribution (Sum of 15d (1), (2), (3) and (4))		▶	70	71
f. Total Distribution (Sum of 15c and 15e)		▶	374	358
g. Copies not Distributed (See Instructions to Publishers #4 (page #3))		▶	89	150
h. Total (Sum of 15f and g)		▶	463	508
i. Percent Paid (15c divided by 15f times 100)		▶	81%	80%

* If you are claiming electronic copies, go to line 16 on page 3. If you are not claiming electronic copies, skip to line 17 on page 3.

16. Electronic Copy Circulation		Average No. Copies Each Issue During Preceding 12 Months	No. Copies of Single Issue Published Nearest to Filing Date
a. Paid Electronic Copies	▶	0	0
b. Total Paid Print Copies (Line 15c) + Paid Electronic Copies (Line 16a)	▶	304	287
c. Total Print Distribution (Line 15f) + Paid Electronic Copies (Line 16a)	▶	374	358
d. Percent Paid (Both Print & Electronic Copies) (16b divided by 16c × 100)	▶	81%	80%

☒ I certify that 50% of all my distributed copies (electronic and print) are paid above a nominal price.

17. Publication of Statement of Ownership

☒ If the publication is a general publication, publication of this statement is required. Will be printed ☐ Publication not required.

in the OCTOBER 2016 issue of this publication.

18. Signature and Title of Editor, Publisher, Business Manager, or Owner	Date
[signature]	9/18/2016

STEPHEN R. BUSHING - INVENTORY DISTRIBUTION CONTROL MANAGER

I certify that all information furnished on this form is true and complete. I understand that anyone who furnishes false or misleading information on this form or who omits material or information requested on the form may be subject to criminal sanctions (including fines and imprisonment) and/or civil sanctions (including civil penalties).

PS Form **3526**, July 2014 (Page 2 of 4)

PRIVACY NOTICE: See our privacy policy on www.usps.com.

Moving?

Make sure your subscription moves with you!

To notify us of your new address, find your **Clinics Account Number** (located on your mailing label above your name), and contact customer service at:

Email: journalscustomerservice-usa@elsevier.com

800-654-2452 (subscribers in the U.S. & Canada)
314-447-8871 (subscribers outside of the U.S. & Canada)

Fax number: 314-447-8029

Elsevier Health Sciences Division
Subscription Customer Service
3251 Riverport Lane
Maryland Heights, MO 63043

*To ensure uninterrupted delivery of your subscription, please notify us at least 4 weeks in advance of move.

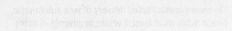

Printed and bound by CPI Group (UK) Ltd, Croydon, CR0 4YY

08/05/2025

01864686-0008